LIGHT ON LIFE

LIGHT ON LIFE

The Yoga Journey to Wholeness, Inner Peace, and Ultimate Freedom

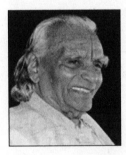

B.K.S. IYENGAR

with John J. Evans and Douglas Abrams

RODALE

Book design by Christina Gaugler

Library of Congress Cataloging-in-Publication Data

Iyengar, B. K. S., date.
    Light on life : the yoga journey to wholeness, inner peace, and ultimate freedom /
B.K.S. Iyengar, with John J. Evans and Douglas Abrams.
        p.   cm.
Includes index.
ISBN-13 978–1–59486–248–9 hardcover
ISBN-10 1–59486–248–6 hardcover
ISBN-13 978–1–59486–524–4 paperback
ISBN-10 1–59486–524–8 paperback
1. Hatha yoga.   2. Spiritual life.   I. Evans, John J.   II. Abrams, Douglas.   III. Title.
B132.Y6I94   2005
294.5'436—dc22   2005015700

Distributed to the trade by Holtzbrinck Publishers

2	4	6	8	10	9	7	5	3	1	hardcover
				10	9					paperback

To find an Iyengar certified teacher, go to WWW.IYNAUS.ORG
OR CALL 800-889-YOGA.

RODALE
LIVE YOUR WHOLE LIFE™

We inspire and enable people to improve their lives and the world around them

For more of our products visit **rodalestore.com** or call 800-848-4735

To my father, Bellur Krishnamachar,

my mother, Seshamma,

and my birthplace, Bellur

Contents

Preface

ix

Introduction: Freedom Awaits

xiii

Chapter 1

The Inward Journey

3

Chapter 2

Stability—The Physical Body (*Asana*)

21

Chapter 3

Vitality—The Energy Body (*Prana*)

65

Chapter 4

Clarity—The Mental Body (*Manas*)

107

Chapter 5

Wisdom—The Intellectual Body (*Vijnana*)

147

Chapter 6

Bliss—The Divine Body (*Ananda*)

187

Chapter 7

Living in Freedom

227

Asanas for Emotional Stability

267

Index

271

Preface

If this book is to lay any claim to authenticity, it must make one point clear above all others. It is this: By persistent and sustained practice, anyone and everyone can make the yoga journey and reach the goal of illumination and freedom. Krishna, Buddha, and Jesus lie in the hearts of all. They are not film stars, mere idols of adulation. They are great inspirational figures whose example is there to be followed. They act as our role models today. Just as they reached Self-Realization, so may we.

Many of you may worry that you are unable to meet the challenges that lie ahead. I want to assure you that you can. I am a man who started from nowhere; I was heavily disadvantaged in many ways. After much time and effort, I began to reach somewhere. I literally emerged from darkness to light, from mortal sickness to health, from crude ignorance to immersion in the ocean of knowledge by one means alone, namely by zealous persistence in the art and science of yoga practice (*sadhana*). What held good for me will hold good for you too.

Today you also have the benefit of many gifted yoga teachers. When I began yoga, there was, I am sorry to say, no wise, kind teacher to lead me. In fact my own Guru refused to answer any of my innocent inquiries on yoga. He did not instruct me as I do my students, offering them step-by-step guidance in an asana. He would simply demand a posture and leave it to me or his other students to figure out how it could be realized. Perhaps that stimulated some stubborn aspect of my nature, which allied to unshakable faith in the subject of yoga made me burn to go on. I am ardent and passionate, and maybe I needed to show the world that I was not worthless. But far more than that, I wanted to find out who I was. I wanted to understand this mysterious and marvelous "yoga," which could reveal to us our innermost secrets, as equally as it revealed those of the universe around us and our place in it as joyful, suffering, puzzled human beings.

I learned through practice, earned a bit of experienced knowledge, and reinvested that knowledge and understanding in order to learn more. By following the right direction and with the help of a naturally sensitive perception, I was able to further my knowledge. This produced in me a growing accumulation of refined experience that eventually revealed the essence of yoga knowledge.

It took me whole decades to appreciate the depth and true value of yoga. Sacred texts supported my discoveries, but it was not they that signposted the way. What I learned through yoga, I found out through yoga. I am not, however, a "self-made man." I am only what seventy-two years of devoted yoga sadhana has created out of me. Any contribution I have made to the world has been the fruit of my sadhana.

This sadhana provided me with the tenacity of purpose to continue even through trying times. My disinclination toward laxer lifestyles kept me on the straight path, but I never shunned anyone, for I have come to see the light of the soul in all. Yoga ferried me across the great river from the bank of ignorance to the shore of knowledge and wisdom. It is no extravagant claim to say that wisdom has come to me by the practice of yoga, and the grace of God has lit the lamp of the inner core in me. This allows me to see that same light of the soul glowing in all other beings.

You, my readers, must understand that you are already starting from somewhere. You have the beginning already shown to you, and no one knows in what wholeness and felicity you may end. If you take up any noble line and stick to it, you can reach the ultimate. Be inspired but not proud. Do not aim low; you will miss the mark. Aim high; you will be on the threshold of bliss.

Patanjali, of whom you will hear much in this book, is considered the father of yoga. In reality as far as we know, he was a yogi and a polymath living around fifth century B.C. India, who collated and elaborated existing knowledge of the yogis' life and practices. He wrote the *Yoga Sutras*, literally a thread of aphorisms about yoga, consciousness, and the human condition. Patanjali also explained the relationship between the natural world and the innermost and transcendent soul. (For those who wish to pursue their textual studies further, I have included references to his great work. See my book *Light on the Yoga Sutras of Patanjali*).

What Patanjali said applies to me and will apply to you. He wrote, "With this truth bearing light will begin a new life. Old unwanted impressions are discarded and we are protected from the damaging effects of new experiences." (*Yoga Sutras*, Chapter I, Verse 50)

It is my hope that my own lowly beginnings and ordinariness may serve as a source of encouragement as you seek this truth and begin a new life. Yoga transformed my life from a parasitic one to a life of purpose. Later yoga inspired me to partake in the joy and nobility of life, which I carried to many thousands of people without consideration of religion, caste, gender, or nationality. I am so grateful for what yoga has made of my life that I have always sought to share it.

In this spirit I offer my experiences through this book in the hope that with faith, love, persistence, and perseverance you will savor the sweet flavor of yoga. Carry the flame forward so that it may bring the blissful light of the knowledge of true reality to future generations.

This book owes its conception and delivery to a number of people who worked together to bring it to its final state so that I may offer it to you. I would like to acknowledge in particular Doug Abrams of Idea Architects, John J. Evans, Geeta S. Iyengar, Uma Dhavale, Stephanie Quirk, Daniel Rivers-Moore, Jackie Wardle, Stephanie Tade, and Chris Potash. My gratitude goes to Rodale for bringing this work to the public at large; I share all credit and merit with them.

Yoga was my Destiny, and for the past seventy years, yoga has been my life, a life fused with the practice, philosophy, and teaching of the art of yoga. Like all destinies, like all great adventures, I have gone to places I never imagined before I set out. For me it has been a journey of discovery. In historical terms it has been one of rediscovery but undertaken from a unique perspective: Innovation within traditional boundaries. These past seventy years have taken me on the Inward Journey toward a vision of the Soul. This book contains my triumphs, struggles, battles, sorrows, and joys.

Fifty years ago, I came to the West to shed Light on Yoga. Now through this book, I am presenting half a century of my experience in order to shed Light on Life. The popularity of yoga and my part in spreading its teaching are a great source of satisfaction to me. But I do not want yoga's widespread popularity to eclipse the depth of what it has to give to the practitioner. Fifty years after my first trip west and after so much devoted yoga practice by so many, I now wish to share with you the whole of the yoga journey.

It is my profound hope that my end can be your beginning.

Introduction: Freedom Awaits

When I left India and came to Europe and America a half century ago, open-mouthed audiences gaped at the presentation of *yogasana* positions, seeing them as some exotic form of contortionism. These very same asanas have now been embraced by many millions of people throughout the world, and their physical and therapeutic benefits are widely acknowledged. This in itself is an extraordinary transformation, as yoga has lit a fire in the hearts of so many.

I set off in yoga seventy years ago when ridicule, rejection, and outright condemnation were the lot of a seeker through yoga even in its native land of India. Indeed, if I had become a *sadhu*, a mendicant holy man, wandering the great trunk roads of British India, begging bowl in hand, I would have met with less derision and won more respect. At one time, I was asked to become a *sannyasin* and renounce the world, but I declined. I wanted to live as an ordinary householder with all the trials and tribulations of life and to take my yoga practice to average people who share with me the common life of work, marriage, and children. I was blessed with all three, including a long and joyous marriage to my beloved late wife, Ramamani, children, and grandchildren.

The life of a householder is difficult, and it always has been. Most of us encounter hardship and suffering, and many are plagued by physical and emotional pain, stress, sadness, loneliness, and anxiety. While we often think of these as the problems caused by the demands of modern life, human life has always had the same hardships and the same challenges—making a living, raising a family, and finding meaning and purpose.

These have always and will always be the challenges that we humans face. As animals, we walk the earth. As bearers of a divine essence, we are among the stars. As human beings, we are caught in the middle, seeking to reconcile the paradox of how to make our way upon the earth while striving for something more permanent and more profound. So many seek this greater Truth in the heavens, but it lies much closer than the clouds. It is within us and can be found by anyone on the Inward Journey.

What most people want is the same. Most people simply want physical and mental health, understanding and wisdom, and peace and freedom. Often our means of pursuing these basic human needs come apart at the seams, as we are pulled by the different and often competing demands of human life. Yoga, as it was understood by its sages, is designed to satisfy all these human needs in a comprehensive, seamless whole. Its goal is nothing less than to attain the integrity of oneness—oneness with ourselves and as a consequence oneness with all that lies beyond ourselves. We become the harmonious microcosm in the universal macrocosm. Oneness, what I often call *integration*, is the foundation for wholeness, inner peace, and ultimate freedom.

Yoga allows you to rediscover a sense of wholeness in your life, where you do not feel like you are constantly trying to fit the broken pieces together. Yoga allows you to find an inner peace that is not ruffled and riled by the endless stresses and struggles of life. Yoga allows you to find a new kind of freedom that you may not have known even existed. To a yogi, freedom implies not being battered by the dualities of life, its ups and downs, its pleasures and its suffering. It implies equanimity and ultimately that there is an inner serene core of one's being that is never out of touch with the unchanging, eternal infinite.

As I have said already, anyone can embark on the Inward Journey. Life itself seeks fulfillment as plants seek the sunlight. The Universe did not create Life in the hope that the failure of the majority would underscore the success of the few. Spiritually at least, we live in a democracy, an equal opportunity society.

Yoga is not meant to be a religion or a dogma for any one culture. While yoga sprang from the soil of India, it is meant as a universal path, a way open to all regardless of their birth and background. Patanjali used the expression *sarvabhauma*—universal—some 2,500 years ago. We are all human beings, but we have been taught to think of ourselves as Westerners or Easterners. If we were left to ourselves, we would simply be individual human beings—no Africans, no Indians, no Europeans, no Americans. Coming from India, I inevitably developed certain Indian characteristics adopted from the culture in which I was nurtured. We all do this. There is no difference in the soul—what I call the "Seer." The difference comes only between the "garments" of the seer—the ideas about our selves that we wear. Break them. Do not feed them with divisive ideas. That is what yoga teaches. When you and I meet together, we forget ourselves—our cultures and classes. There are no divisions, and we talk mind to mind, soul to soul. We are no different in our deepest needs. We are all human.

Yoga recognizes that the way our bodies and minds work has changed very little over the millennia. The way we function inside our skin is not susceptible to differ either in time or from place to place. In the functioning of our minds, in our way of relating to each other, there are inherent stresses, like geological fault lines that, left unaddressed, will always cause things to go wrong, whether individually or collectively. The whole thrust of the yogic philosophical and scientific inquiry has therefore been to examine the nature of being, with a view to learning to respond to the stresses of life without so many tremors and troubles.

Yoga does not look on greed, violence, sloth, excess, pride, lust, and fear as ineradicable forms of original sin that exist to wreck our happiness—or indeed on which to found our happiness. They are seen as natural, if unwelcome, manifestations of the human disposition and predicament that are to be solved, not suppressed or denied. Our flawed mechanisms of perception and thought are not a cause for grief (though they bring us grief), but an opportunity to evolve, for an internal evolution of consciousness that will also make possible in a sustainable form our aspirations toward what we call individual success and global progress.

Yoga is the rule book for playing the game of Life, but in this game no one needs to lose. It is tough, and you need to train hard. It requires the willingness to think for yourself, to observe and correct, and to surmount occasional setbacks. It demands honesty, sustained application, and above all love in your heart. If you are interested to understand what it means to be a human being, placed between earth and sky, if you are interested in where you come from and where you will be able to go, if you want happiness and long for freedom, then you have already begun to take the first steps toward the journey inward.

The rules of nature cannot be bent. They are impersonal and implacable. But we do play with them. By accepting nature's challenge and joining the game, we find ourselves on a windswept and exciting journey that will pay benefits commensurate to the time and effort we put in—the lowest being our ability to tie our own shoelaces when we are eighty and the highest being the opportunity to taste the essence of life itself.

My Yogic Journey

Most of those who begin to practice yogasana, the poses of yoga, do so for practical and often physical reasons. Perhaps it is for some medical problem such as a bad back, a sports injury, high blood pressure, or arthritis. Or perhaps it is as a result of a broader concern to do with achieving a better lifestyle or coping with stress, weight problems, or addiction. Very few people begin yoga because they believe it will be a way to achieve spiritual enlightenment, and indeed a good number may be quite skeptical about the whole idea of spiritual self-realization. Actually, this is not a bad thing because it means most of the people who come to yoga are practical people who have practical problems and aims—people who are grounded in the ways and means of life, people who are sensible.

When I set off in yoga, I also had no understanding of the greater glory of yoga. I too was seeking its physical benefits, and it was these that truly saved my life. When I say that yoga saved my life, I am not exaggerating. It was yoga that gave me a new birth with health from illness and firmness from infirmity.

At the time of my birth, in December 1918, India, like so many countries, was devastated by a major world epidemic of influenza. My mother, Sheshamma, was herself in the grip of the disease at the time when she was pregnant with me, and as a result, I was born very sickly. My arms were thin, my legs were spindly, and my stomach protruded in an ungainly manner. So frail was I, in fact, that I was not expected to survive. My head used to hang down, and I had to lift it with great effort. My head was disproportionately large to the rest of my body, and my brothers and sisters often teased me. I was the eleventh child of thirteen, although only ten survived.

This frailty and sickliness remained with me throughout my early years. As a boy, I suffered from numerous ailments, including frequent bouts of malaria, typhoid, and tuberculosis. My poor health was matched, as it often is when one is sick, by my poor mood. A deep melancholy often overtook me, and at times I asked myself whether life was worth the trouble of living.

I grew up in the village of Bellur in the Kolar District of the southern Indian state of Karnataka, a small farming community of some 500 people, making a living by cultivating rice, millet, and a few vegetables. My family was better off than many, however, since my father had inherited a small plot of land and also drew a State salary for acting as a schoolmaster in a somewhat larger village a short distance away. Bellur itself did not at the time have a school of its own.

When I was five years old, my family moved from Bellur to Bangalore. My father had suffered from appendicitis since he was a child and had not received any treatment for it. Shortly before my ninth birthday, the appendicitis, which had flared up once again, proved fatal. From his sick bed, my father called me and told me that he would die when I was nearing nine as his father had died when he was nearing nine. He also told me that he had struggled very hard in his youth and that I would struggle very hard in mine, but eventually I would lead a happy life. I daresay my father's prophecy came true both in the struggle and in the happiness. At the time a great vacuum was left in my family, and there was no strong guiding hand to help me through my sickness and my schooling. As often as not, I missed school through illness, and I fell behind in my studies.

Despite my father's being a schoolteacher, my family were Brahmins—members of the priestly caste in India who are born to a life of religious duty. Typically, a Brahmin will earn a living through offerings made by people, through payment for the performance of religious ceremonies, and perhaps through the patronage of a wealthy or aristocratic family or individual. In accordance with Indian tradition, Brahmins generally marry into other Brahmin families, through arranged marriages. And so my sister was given in marriage at the age of eleven to a distant relative of ours, Shriman T. Krishnamacharya. This was an excellent match, as he was a venerable and revered scholar of both philosophy and Sanskrit. After completing his academic studies, Krishnamacharya had spent many further years in the Himalayan Mountains near the border of Nepal with Tibet, pursuing the study of yoga under the tutelage of Shri Ramamohana Brahmachari.

At this time, Maharajas, Indian Kings, lived in great fortresses, riding out on their elephants to hunt tigers in personal fiefdoms larger than many European countries. The Maharaja of Mysore heard of my brother-in-law's scholarship and prowess in yoga and took a great interest in him. The Maharaja invited my brother-in-law to teach in his Sanskrit college, and later to set up a school of yoga, at his magnificent Jaganmohan Palace. The Maharaja would from time to time also ask Krishnamacharya to travel to other cities to spread the message of yoga to a broader public. It was during one such journey in 1934, when I was some fourteen years old, that my brother-in-law asked me to come from Bangalore to Mysore and spend some time with his wife (my sister) and her family while he was away. On my brother-in-law's return, when I asked to be allowed to go back to my mother and to my other brothers and sisters, he proposed instead that I should stay in Mysore working on yoga to improve my health.

Seeing that the general state of my health was so poor, my brother-in-law recommended a stiff regime of yoga practice to knock me into shape and strengthen me up to face life's trials and challenges as I approached adulthood. If my brother-in-law also had an eye to my deeper spiritual or personal development, he did not say so at the time. The situation seemed right and the time propitious, and I embarked upon my training at my brother-in-law's yoga school.

This was to be the major turning point in my life—the moment when destiny came to meet me, and I had the opportunity to embrace it or to turn away. Like for so many people, these pivotal moments pass with no great fanfare, but instead become the starting point for years of steady work and growth. So it was that my brother-in-law, Shriman T. Krishnamacharya, became my revered teacher and guru and took the place of my mother and late father as my effective guardian.

One of the duties I was often called upon to perform during this period of my life was to give demonstrations of yoga for the Maharaja's court and for visiting dignitaries and guests. It was my guru's duty to provide for the edification and amusement of the Maharaja's entourage by putting his students—of whom I was one of the youngest—through their paces and showing off their ability to stretch and bend their bodies into the most impressive and astonishing postures. I pushed myself to the limits in my practice in order to do my duty to my teacher and guardian and to satisfy his demanding expectations.

At eighteen, I was sent to Pune to spread the teaching of yoga. There I did not possess the language nor have community, family, friends, or even safe employment. At the time all I had was my practice of asana, of yoga postures—not even the breathing practices of *pranayama*, not texts, not yoga philosophy.

I embarked on the practice of asana as a man might set off to sail the world in a craft he could barely handle, clinging to it for dear life and finding only solace from the stars. Although I knew that others had sailed the world before me, I did not have their maps. It was a voyage of discovery. In time I came across some maps, usually charted some hundreds or thousands of years before, and found that my discoveries corresponded with and confirmed theirs. I continued, heartened and encouraged, to see if I too could make their distant landfalls and better learn how to handle my ship. I wanted precisely to chart every coastline, measure the depth of every sea, happen on beautiful unknown islands, and record each perilous hidden reef or tidal current that threatens our navigation of the ocean of life.

In this way, body became my first instrument to know what yoga is. The slow process of refinement started then and continues in my practice to this day. In the process yogasana brought tremendous physical benefits and helped me to grow from a sickly child into a reasonably fit and agile young man. My own body was the laboratory, in which I saw the health benefits of yoga, but I could already see that yoga would have as many benefits for my head and heart as it did for my body. It would be impossible to overestimate the gratitude I bear to this great subject that saved and uplifted me.

Your Yogic Journey

This book is about Life. It is an attempt to light the way for you and other spiritual seekers. It aims to map out a path that all may follow. It offers advice, methods, and a philosophical framework at a level that even a newcomer to the practice of yoga may grasp. It does not offer shortcuts or vain promises to the gullible. It has taken me more than seventy years of constant application to reach where I am today. That does not mean that you need seventy years to reap the rewards of yoga practice. Yoga brings gifts from your very first day. These benefits can be experienced even by raw beginners, who feel something beginning to happen at a deep level in their bodies, in their minds, and even in their souls. Some describe the first gifts as a new feeling of lightness or calm or joy.

The miracle is that after seventy years, these gifts are still increasing for me. The benefits of practice cannot always be anticipated. When they come, it is so often as unexpected bounty in forms one had not expected. But if you think that learning to touch your toes or even stand on your head is the whole of yoga, you have missed most of its bounty, most of its blessings, and most of its beauty.

Yoga releases the creative potential of Life. It does this by establishing a structure for self-realization, by showing how we can progress along the journey, and by opening a sacred vision of the Ultimate, of our Divine Origin, and final Destiny. The Light that yoga sheds on Life is something special. It is transformative. It does not just change the way we see things; it transforms the person who sees. It brings knowledge and elevates it to wisdom.

The Light on Life we envisage here is unadulterated insight, pure truth (*satya*), which, allied to non-violence, was the guiding principle of Mahatma Gandhi and changed the world for all its inhabitants.

Socrates admonished one to know thy self. To know oneself is to know one's body, mind, and soul. Yoga, I often say, is like music. The rhythm of the body, the melody of the mind, and the harmony of the soul create the symphony of life. The Inward Journey will allow you to explore and to integrate each of these aspects of your being. From your physical body, you will journey inward to discover your "subtle bodies"—your energy body, where breath and emotions reside; your mental body, where thoughts and obsessions can be mastered; your intellectual body, where intelligence and wisdom can be found; and your divine body, where the Universal Soul can be glimpsed. In the next chapter, we will understand this ancient yogic mapping of the layers of our being. Before we will look at each layer in its own chapter, we must first deepen our understanding of this Inward Journey and how it incorporates the traditional eight limbs or petals of yoga. We must also come to see the relationship between nature and soul; yoga does not reject one for the other but sees them as inseparably joined like earth and sky are joined on the horizon.

You do not need to seek freedom in some distant land, for it exists within your own body, heart, mind, and soul. Illuminated emancipation, freedom, unalloyed and untainted bliss await you, but you must choose to embark on the Inward Journey to discover it.

LIGHT ON LIFE

Parivrtta Janu Sirsasana

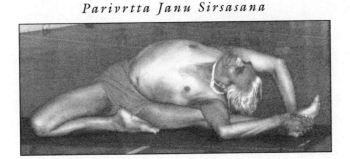

Chapter 1

The Inward Journey

Spiritual realization is the aim that exists in each one of us to seek our divine core. That core, though never absent from anyone, remains latent within us. It is not an outward quest for a Holy Grail that lies beyond, but an Inward Journey to allow the inner core to reveal itself.

In order to find out how to reveal our innermost Being, the sages explored the various sheaths of existence, starting from body and progressing through mind and intelligence, and ultimately to soul. The yogic journey guides us from our periphery, the body, to the center of our being, the soul. The aim is to integrate the various layers so that the inner divinity shines out as through clear glass.

Kosas—The Sheaths of Being

Yoga identifies five of these different levels or sheaths of being (*kosas*), which must be completely integrated and in harmony with each other in order for us to achieve wholeness. When these subtle sheaths are in disharmony, they become sullied like a mirror reflecting the tarnished images of the sensory and sensual world. The mirror reflects what is in the world around us rather than letting the clear light of the soul within shine out. It is then that we experience disease and despair. True health requires not only the effective functioning of the physical exterior of our being, but also the vitality, strength, and sensitivity of the subtle levels within.

Most of us think of our "body" as simply our physical form—our skin, bones, muscles, and internal organs. For yoga, however, this is only the outermost layer of our body or *annamaya kosa*. It is this anatomical body that encompasses the other four subtle bodies, or kosas.

The kosas are like the layers of an onion or the Russian dolls where one is nested within the other. These include our energetic body (*pranamaya kosa*), our mental body (*manomaya kosa*), our intellectual body (*vijnanamaya kosa*), and ultimately our blissful or soul body (*anandamaya kosa*). When these bodies or sheaths are misaligned or clash with one another, we inevitably encounter the alienation and fragmentation that so trouble our world. When, on the other hand, we are able to bring the various sheaths of our body into alignment and harmony with one another, the fragmentation disappears, integration is achieved, and unity is established. The physical body (annamaya kosa) must connect with and thereby imprint upon the energetic and organic body (pranamaya kosa), which must, in turn, accord with the mental body (manomaya kosa), the mental body with the intellectual body (vijnanamaya kosa), and the intellectual body with the blissful body (anandamaya kosa). Likewise, if there is no communication between the blissful body and the physical body, then the blissful body cannot bring its illumination to the motion and action of the physical body, and there is darkness in life and not Light on Life.

The demarcation of the different sheaths is essentially hypothetical. We are unique and integral. Nevertheless, in order to achieve the integrity and wholeness we desire, there must be communication from the inner to the outer and the outer to the inner as each sheath blends with the next. Only then are we bound together as one functional human being. If not, we experience dissolution and fragmentation, which make life uncomfortable and confusing.

It is essential for the follower of the yoga journey to understand the need for integration and balance in the kosa. For example, the mental and intellectual bodies (manomaya and vijnanamaya kosa) must function effectively in order for us to observe, analyze, and reflect what is happening in the physical and energetic bodies (annamaya and pranamaya kosa) and make readjustments.

The physical body in other words is not something separate from our mind and soul. We are not supposed to neglect or deny our body as some ascetics suggest. Nor are we to become fixated on our body—our mortal self—either. The aim of yoga is to discover our immortal Self. The practice of yoga teaches us to live fully—physically and spiritually—by cultivating each of the various sheaths.

I hope as you read on you will begin to understand that if you too live and practice yoga in the right way and with the right attitude, far greater benefits and more radical changes will take place than mere physical flexibility. There is no progress toward ultimate freedom without transformation, and this is the key issue in all people's lives, whether they practice yoga or not. If we can understand how our mind and heart works, we have a chance to answer the question, "Why do I keep making the same old mistakes?"

It is the map the ancients left us that gives us the form for the chapters of this book. Their knowledge and technology make up the contents. The human being is a continuum—there are no tangible frontiers between the kosas as there are no frontiers between body, mind, and soul. But for convenience sake, and to aid us on our journey, yoga describes us in terms of these discrete layers. We should imagine them as blending from one into the other like the colors of the rainbow. Following this traditional description of the five different bodies or kosas, we have divided this discussion into five central chapters of "Stability: The Physical Body" (annamaya kosa), "Vitality: The Energy Body" (pranamaya kosa), "Clarity: The Mental Body" (manomaya kosa), "Wisdom: The Intellectual Body" (vijnanamaya kosa), and "Bliss: The Divine Body" (anandamaya kosa).

In these chapters we discuss the various stages of the Inward Journey as we discover Nature (*prakrti*), which includes the physical body, and Soul (*purusa*). As we explore the Soul, it is important to remember that this exploration will take place within Nature (the body), for that is where we are and what we are. Our specific field of exploration is ourselves, from skin to unknown center. Yoga is concerned with this fusion of nature and soul because this is the essence of human life with all of its challenges, contradictions, and joys.

Living between Earth and Sky

As I have said, we human beings live between the two realities of earth and sky. The earth stands for all that is practical, material, tangible, and incarnate. It is the knowable world, objectively knowable through voyages of discovery and observation. We all partake of this world and its knowledge through the vast store of accumulated collective experience. There is one word for all this. It is Nature. In Sanskrit, Nature is called Prakrti. It is composed of five elements, which we characterize as earth, water, fire, air, and space (previously called ether). Consequently and sympathetically, the body is made up of these same five elements, which is why we also use the term prakrti for the body. When space explorers bring back rocks from the moon and scientists study them, they are studying Nature. When we calculate the temperature on the surface of the sun, we are observing Nature. Whether we study planetary Nature or cosmic Nature, it is Nature. Such study is endlessly fascinating because Nature is full of variety. Not only is it full of variety, it is also constantly changing, so there is always something new to see. We too are part of Nature, therefore constantly changing, so we are always looking at Nature from a different viewpoint. We are a little piece of continual change looking at an infinite quantity of continual change. Small wonder that it gets quite exciting. The most important thing we can learn about Nature is the inherent and innate laws by which it functions.

Even hundreds of years before Patanjali wrote the *Yoga Sutras*, Indian yogis were trying to see some pattern in the seemingly chaotic fluctuations of Nature. The infinite variety of natural phenomena gives an appearance of chaos, but, they asked, is it possible that the laws that govern the unending turbulence of nature are orderly and comprehensible? And if we can grasp how they work, would it not be possible for us to emerge from chaos into order? All games are meaningless if you do not know the rules. When you do, they can become very good fun. You still take a few knocks and lose a few games, but at least you are participating; you are playing the game. Yoga says you are playing the game with the body and self. By playing you can learn the rules, and if you observe them, you have a far better chance of success in life as well as of gaining illumination and freedom.

So humankind stands with its feet planted squarely on the earth, as in *Tadasana* (mountain pose), and its head in the sky. But what then do we mean by the sky? Clearly I do not mean the earth's biosphere, or anywhere that physically exists, however far away. I could have said, "Our feet on the earth and our head in the heavens." Many languages do not have two separate words for sky and heaven as English does. The word heaven is useful as it suggests something that is not physical. This opens up possibilities: a) that it is perfect, as nothing physical can be perfect since all phenomena are unstable; b) that it is Universal—i.e. One, whereas Nature is many as we see from its diversity; c) that it is Everywhere, Omnipresent since, not being physical, it is not limited or defined by location; d) that it is supremely Real or Eternal. In yoga the body is held to be of real substance, whereas the changing of ourselves and unveiling of the immeasurable sky within is called *cit-akasha*, or literally the vision of space itself.

Anything physical is always changing, therefore its reality is not constant, not Eternal. Nature is in this sense like an actor who has only different roles. It never takes off its costume and makeup and goes home, but just changes from one role to another, for ever and ever. So with Nature we never quite know where we are, especially as we too are part of it.

The non-physical Reality, however difficult to grasp, must have the advantage of being eternal, always the same. This has a consequence. Whatever is real and unchanging must offer us a fixed point, an orientation, like a perfect north on a compass. And how does a compass work? By an attraction between magnetic north and a magnet in our compass. The compass is ourselves. So we are able to infer that there is a Universal Reality in ourselves that aligns us with a Universal Reality that is everywhere else. Do not forget the word align. It is through the alignment of my body that I discovered the alignment of my mind, self, and intelligence. Alignment from the outermost body or sheath (kosa) to the innermost is the way to bring our own personal Reality into contact with Universal Reality. The Vastasutra Upanishad says, "Setting the limbs along proper lines is praised like the knowledge of Brahman (God)." Even earlier, from the Rig Veda comes, "Every form is an image of the original form." We have seen that this Reality is not changeable in Time or limited by Space. It is free of both. It follows that, although our journey takes place in time and space, if ever we reach its end and encounter the supreme non-physical reality, it will not be in time and space as we know them.

Universal Soul (*Purusa*) and Nature (*Prakrti*)

I have purposely avoided until now using the usual translation for the non-physical reality as its mention usually stops people thinking for themselves. In Sanskrit, the word is Purusa. In English we can call it Cosmic or Universal Soul. The word Soul usually has such strong religious connotations that people either accept or dismiss it without reflection. They forget that it is simply our word for an abiding reality. It is logical but remains conceptual to our minds until we experience its realization within ourselves.

We rightly associate this abiding reality with selfless love, which is founded in the perception of unity, not difference. The strength of a mother's love derives from her unity with the child. In unity there is no possession, as possession is a dual state, containing me and it. Soul is unchanging, eternal, and constant; it always remains as witness, rooted in divine origin and oneness. The whole practice of yoga is concerned with exploring the relationship between Prakrti and Purusa, between Nature and Soul. It is about, to return to our original image, learning to live between the earth and the sky. That is the human predicament, our joy and our woe, our salvation or our downfall. Nature and Soul are mingled together. Some would say they are married. It is through the correct practice of asana and *pranayama* and the other petals of yoga that the practitioner (*sadhaka*) experiences the communication and connection between them. To an average person it might seem that the marriage of Nature and Soul is one of strife and mutual incomprehension. But by communing with them both, they come closer to each other for the purpose of a blessed union. That union removes the veil of ignorance that covers our intelligence. To achieve this union, the sadhaka has to look both within as well as looking out to the frame of the soul, the body. He has to grasp an underlying law or else he will remain in Nature's thrall and Soul will remain merely a concept. Everything that exists in the macrocosm is to be found existing in the microcosm or individual.

The Eight Petals of Yoga

There are eight petals of yoga that reveal themselves progressively to the practitioner. These are external, ethical disciplines (*yama*), internal ethical observances (*niyama*), poses (asana), breath control (pranayama), sensory control and withdrawal (*pratyahara*), concentration (*dharana*), meditation (*dhyana*), and blissful absorption (*samadhi*). We call these the petals of yoga as they join together like the petals of a lotus flower to form one beautiful whole.

As we journey through the interior sheaths (kosa) of the body, from the exterior skin to the innermost self, we will encounter and explore each of the eight petals or stages of yoga described in the *Yoga Sutras*. For the seeker of Truth, these stages remain as important today as they were in the days of Patanjali. We cannot hope to understand and harmonize the sheaths without the precepts and practices provided in the eight petals. I will mention them here briefly, but they will be discussed more fully in the following chapters.

The yoga journey begins with the five universal moral commandments (yama). We learn in this way to develop control over our actions in the external world. The journey continues with five steps of self-purification (niyama). These relate to our inner world and senses of perception and help us to develop self-discipline. We will discuss these throughout the book, but initially they serve to curb our behavior toward others and toward ourselves. These ethical precepts are always with us from the beginning to the end of the yoga journey, for the demonstration of one's spiritual realization lies in none other than how one walks among and interacts with one's fellow human beings.

After all, the goal of yoga may be the ultimate freedom but even before this is achieved, there is an incremental experience of greater freedom as we discover ever more self-control, sensitivity, and awareness that permit us to live the life we aspire to, one of decency; clean, honest human relations; goodwill and fellowship; trust; self-reliance; joy in the fortune of others; and equanimity in the face of our own misfortune. From a state of human goodness, we can progress toward the greater freedom. From doubt, confusion, and vice we cannot. Progression in yoga is a moral one for a very practical reason rather than a judgmental one. It is almost impossible to jump from "bad" to "best" without passing through "good." Also, as ignorance recedes, "good" is an infinitely more comfortable place to be than "bad." What we call "bad" is ignorance in action and, as a strategy for life, thrives only in darkness.

The third petal of yoga is the practice of postures (*yogasana*), which will be the next chapter of this book. Asana maintains the strength and health of the body, without which little progress can be made. It also keeps the body in harmony with nature. We all know that mind affects body, for example, "You look down in the dumps," or "He was crestfallen." Why not, suggests yoga, try the other way round—access mind through body. "Chin up" and "Shoulders back, stand up straight" express this approach. Self-cultivation through asana is the broad gateway leading to the inner enclosures we need to explore. In other words, we are going to try to use asana to sculpt the mind. We must discover what each sheath of being longs for and nourish it according to its subtle appetites. After all, it is the inner or subtler kosa that support the layers exterior to them. So we would say in yoga that the subtle precedes the gross, or spirit precedes matter. But yoga says we must deal with the outer or most manifest first, i.e. legs, arms, spine, eyes, tongue, touch, in order to develop the sensitivity to move inward. This is why asana opens the whole spectrum of yoga's possibilities. There can be no realization of existential, divine bliss without the support of the soul's incarnate vehicle, the food-and-water-fed body, from bone to brain. If we can become aware of its limitations and compulsions, we can transcend them. We all possess some awareness of ethical behavior, but in order to pursue yama and niyama at deeper levels, we must cultivate the mind. We need contentment, tranquility, dispassion, and unselfishness, qualities that have to be earned. It is asana that teaches us the physiology of these virtues.

The fourth petal of yoga concerns the breathing techniques or pranayama (*prana* = vital or cosmic energy, *ayama* = extension, expansion). Breath is the vehicle of consciousness and so, by its slow, measured observation and distribution, we learn to tug our attention away from external desires (*vasana*) toward a judicious, intelligent awareness (*prajna*). As breath stills mind, our energies are free to unhook from the senses and bend inward to pursue the inner quest with heightened, dynamic awareness. Pranayama is not performed by the power of will. The breath must be enticed or cajoled, like catching a horse in a field, not by chasing after it, but by standing still with an apple in one's hand. In this way, pranayama teaches humility and frees us from greed or hankering after the fruits of our actions. Nothing can be forced; receptivity is everything.

The withdrawal of the senses into the mind (pratyahara) is the fifth petal of yoga, also called the hinge of the outer and inner quest. Unfortunately, we misuse our senses, our memories, and our intelligence. We let the potential energies of all these flow outward and get scattered. We may say that we want to reach the domain of the soul, but there remains a great tug-of-war. We neither go in nor out, and that saps the energy. We can do better.

By drawing our senses of perception inward, we are able to experience the control, silence, and quietness of the mind. This ability to still and gently silence the mind is essential, not only for meditation and the inward journey but also so that the intuitive intelligence can function usefully and in a worthwhile manner in the external world.

The final three petals or stages are concentration (dharana), meditation (dhyana), and total absorption (samadhi). These three are a crescendo, the yoga of final integration (*samyama yoga*).

We begin with concentration. Because dharana is so easy to translate as concentration, we often overlook or dismiss it. At school we learn to pay attention. This is useful, but it is not in yogic terms concentration. We do not say of a deer in the forest, "Look, he's concentrating." The deer is in a state of total vibrant awareness in every cell of his body. We often fool ourselves that we are concentrating because we fix our attention on wavering objects—a football match, a film, a novel, the waves of the sea, or a candle flame—but is not even the flame flickering? True concentration is an unbroken thread of awareness. Yoga is about how the Will, working with intelligence and the self-reflexive consciousness, can free us from the inevitability of the wavering mind and outwardly directed senses. Here, asana serves us greatly.

Consider the challenge of body on mind in an asana. The outer leg overstretches, but the inner leg drops. We can choose whether to let the situation be, or we can challenge the imbalance by the application of cognitive comparison supported by the force of will. Maintaining the equilibrium so that there is no back-sliding, we can add our observation of the knees, feet, skin, ankles, soles of feet, toes, etc.; the list is endless. Our attention not only envelopes but penetrates. Can we, like a juggler, keep these many balls in the air without letting any one drop, without release of attention? Is it any wonder asana takes many years to perfect?

When each new point has been studied, adjusted, and sustained, one's awareness and concentration will necessarily be simultaneously directed to myriad points so that in effect consciousness itself is diffused evenly throughout the body. Here consciousness is penetrating and enveloping, illuminated by a directed flow of intelligence and serving as a transformative witness to body and mind. This is a sustained flow of concentration (dharana) leading to an exalted awareness. The ever-alert Will adjusts and refines, creating a totally self-correcting mechanism. In this way, the practice of asana, performed with the involvement of all elements of our being, awakens and sharpens intelligence until it is integrated with our senses, our mind, our memory, our consciousness, and our soul. All of our bones, flesh, joints, fibers, ligaments, senses, mind, and intelligence are harnessed. The self is both the perceiver and the doer. When I use the word "self" with a small s, I mean the totality of our awareness of who and what we are in a natural state of consciousness. Thus the self assumes its natural form, neither bloated nor shrunken. In a perfect asana, performed meditatively and with a sustained current of concentration, the self assumes its perfect form, its integrity being beyond reproach.

If you want a simple way to remember the relationship between asana and concentration (dharana), it is this: If you learn a lot of little things, one day you may end up knowing a big thing.

Next we come to meditation (dhyana). In the speed of modern life, there is an unavoidable undertone of stress. This stress on mind builds up mental disturbances, such as anger and desire, which in turn build up emotional stress. Contrary to what many teachers try to tell you, meditation is not going to remove stress. Meditation is only possible when one has already achieved a certain "stressless" state. To be stressless, the brain must already be calm and cool. By learning how to relax the brain, one can begin to remove stress.

Meditation does not achieve this. You need to achieve all these as a foundation for meditation. However, I am aware that in modern English usage, the word meditation is often used for various forms of stress management and reduction. In this book, I shall be using it in its purest yogic sense as the seventh petal, which can be achieved only when all other physical and mental weaknesses have largely been eliminated. Technically speaking, true meditation in the yogic sense cannot be done by a person who is under stress or who has a weak body, weak lungs, hard muscles, collapsed spine, fluctuating mind, mental agitation, or timidity. Often people think that sitting quietly is meditation. This is a misunderstanding. True meditation leads us to wisdom (*jnana*) and awareness (prajna), and this specifically helps in understanding that we are more than our ego. For this one needs the preparations of the postures and the breathing, the withdrawal of the senses and concentration.

This process of relaxing the brain is achieved through asana. We generally think of mind as being in our head. In asana our consciousness spreads throughout the body, eventually diffusing in every cell, creating a complete awareness. In this way stressful thought is drained away, and our mind focuses on the body, intelligence, and awareness as a whole.

This allows the brain to be more receptive, and concentration becomes natural. How to keep the brain cells in a relaxed, receptive, and concentrated state is the art that yoga teaches. You must also remember that meditation (dhyana) is part and parcel of yoga; it is not separate. Yama, niyama, asana, pranayama, pratyahara, dharana, dhyana, and samadhi, all these are the petals of yoga. There is meditation in everything. Indeed, in all these petals of yoga one needs a reflective or a meditative mood.

The stress that saturates the brain is decreased through asana and pranayama, so the brain is rested, and there is a release from strain. Similarly, while doing the various types of pranayama the whole body is irrigated with energy. To practice pranayama people must have strength in their muscles and nerves, concentration and persistence, determination and endurance. These are all learned through the practice of asana. The nerves are soothed, the brain is calmed, and the hardness and rigidity of the lungs are loosened. The nerves are helped to remain healthy. You are at once one with yourself, and that is meditation.

One way of looking at meditation was offered by the Israeli astronaut, Ilan Ramon, who was killed in the Columbia Space Shuttle. After circling the earth, he made an appeal for "peace and a better life for everyone on earth." He was not the only astronaut to experience this transcendent vision. Others noted that "having seen earth from a vantage point that blurs political difference, people who travel in space share a unique perspective." Yet they are looking down on a planet where violent struggle is the norm. There is the biblical phrase "an eye for an eye," a philosophy of revenge, not justice. But Mahatma Gandhi warned that in a world ruled by an eye for an eye, soon the whole world will be blind.

We cannot all go into outer space to glimpse a planet where shared human goals can be achieved by peaceful cooperation. But when we look at photos of our blue orb hanging in space with no national boundaries cut into its surface and the white cloak of clouds enveloping it, we too are moved by the earth's unity. How then do we live this unity? Duality is the seed of conflict. But we all have access to a space, an inner space, where there is an end to duality, an end to conflict. This is what meditation teaches us, the cessation of the impersonating ego and the dawn of the true, unified Self, beyond which there is no other. Yoga says that the highest experience of freedom is Oneness, the supreme reality of unity. But we cannot penetrate inward in order to experience immortal bliss without first harmonizing the five sheaths that encompass the soul.

Asana and pranayama are the apprenticeship to that transcendence of duality. Not only do they prepare our bodies, spine, and breath for the challenge of inner serenity, but Patanjali specifically said that asana teaches us to transcend duality, that is, hot and cold, honor and dishonor, wealth and poverty, loss and gain. Asana bestows the firmness to live with equanimity in the vicissitudes of the world's hurly-burly. Although it is strictly speaking possible only to meditate in one asana, it is possible to perform all asana in a meditative way, and this is what my practice has now become. My asana is meditative, and my practice of pranayama is devotional. Meditation itself is the final conquest and dissolution of the ego, the false self, which impersonates the Real Self. Once duality is reconciled and transcended, by the grace of God, the supreme gift of samadhi may be granted.

In the final stage of samadhi (union), the individual self, with all its attributes, merges with the Divine Self, with the Universal Spirit. Yogis realize that the divine is not more heavenward than inward and in this final quest of the soul, seekers become seers. In this way they experience the divine at the core of their being. Samadhi is usually described as the final freedom, freedom from the wheel of *karma*, of cause and effect, action and reaction. Samadhi has nothing to do with perpetuating our mortal self. Samadhi is an opportunity to encounter our imperishable Self before the transient vehicle of body disappears, as in the cycle of nature, it surely must.

Yogis, however, do not stay in this stage of exalted bliss, but when they return to the world their actions are different, as they know in their innermost being that the divine unites us all and that a word or action done to another is ultimately done equally to oneself. Yoga considers actions to be of four kinds: black—those that bring only ill consequences; grey—those whose effects are mixed; white—those that bring good results; and a fourth, those that are without color, in which action brings no reaction. These last are the deeds of the enlightened yogi, who can act in the world without further chaining himself to the karmic wheel of becoming, or causality. Even white actions, consciously performed with good intent, bind us to a future in which we must harvest the good results. An example of a white action might be that if a lawyer, for the sake of justice, were to struggle to save an innocent man who is wrongly accused. But if a child were to dash into the road in front of an oncoming car, and you, in a flash, without a second's reflection, snatched the child out of harm's way, it would be like a yogi's action, that is to say, one based on direct, instantaneous perception and action. You would not congratulate yourself by saying, "How well I saved that child." That's because you would not feel yourself to be the author, but rather the instrument of something that was simply "right," existing purely in the moment, without reference to past or future.

For this reason, the final chapter in this book, "Living in Freedom," concerns ethics and returns to the first two stages of yoga (yama and niyama). By seeing how the free or self-realized man or woman lives in the world, we will see what we can learn for how each of us lives not at some ultimate destination but each step along the journey inward and the journey of life onward.

Learning to Live in the Natural World

Before beginning this journey inward, we must clarify its nature. There is a frequent misunderstanding of the journey inward or the spiritual path, which suggests to most people a rejection of the natural world, the mundane, the practical, the pleasurable. On the contrary, to a yogi (or indeed a Taoist master or Zen monk) the path toward spirit lies entirely in the domain of nature. It is the exploration of nature from the world of appearances, or surface, into the subtlest heart of living matter. Spirituality is not some external goal that one must seek but a part of the divine core of each of us, which we must reveal. For the yogi, spirit is not separate from body. Spirituality, as I have tried to make clear, is not ethereal and outside nature but accessible and palpable in our very own bodies. Indeed the very idea of a spiritual path is a misnomer. After all, how can you move *toward* something that, like Divinity, is already by definition everywhere? A better image might be that if we tidy and clean our houses enough, we might one day notice that Divinity has been sitting in them all along. We do the same with the sheaths of the body, polishing them until they become a pure window to the divine.

A scientist sets out to conquer nature through knowledge—external nature, external knowledge. By these means he may split the atom and achieve external power. A yogi sets out to explore his own internal nature, to penetrate the atom (*atma*) of being. He does not gain dominion over wide lands and restless seas, but over his own recalcitrant flesh and febrile mind. This is the power of compassionate truth. The presence of truth can make us feel naked, but compassion takes all our shame away. It is this inner quest for growth and evolution, or "involution," that is the profound and transformational yogic journey that awaits the seeker after Truth. We begin this involution with what is most tangible, our physical body, and the yogasana practice helps us to understand and learn how to play this magnificent instrument that each of us has been given.

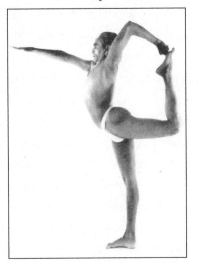

Chapter 2

STABILITY
The Physical Body (*Asana*)

It is here that the yogi embarks on the inward journey toward the core of his being. Many associate yoga with a rejection of the world, its responsibilities, and commitments, and with extreme austerity leading even to self-mortification. But is not the greater challenge and greater fulfillment to be found living in the world with its tribulations and temptations, and at the same time to maintain both balance and self-control in the everyday life of a householder? To be spiritual, one must not deny or forget the body. Throughout the journey to the spiritual goal, the body must be kept active. Yoga is as old and traditional as civilization, yet it persists in modern society as a means to achieving essential vitality. But yoga demands that we develop not only strength in body but attention and awareness in mind. The yogi knows that the physical body is not only the temple for our soul but the means by which we embark on the inward journey toward the core. Only by first attending to the physical body can we hope to accomplish anything in our spiritual lives. If a man or woman has aspirations to experience the divine, but his or her body is too weak to bear the burden, of what use are their aspirations and ambitions? That's all the more reason, therefore, for the vast majority of us who suffer from physical limitations and debilities to some degree to start yoga as soon as possible so that we may fit ourselves for the journey ahead of us.

Yoga offers us techniques to become aware, to expand and penetrate, and to change and evolve in order to become competent in the lives we live and to initiate sensitivity and receptivity toward the life of which we are still only dimly aware. We begin at the level of the physical body, the aspect of ourselves that is most concrete and accessible to all of us. It is here that *yogasana* and *pranayama* practice allow us to understand our body with ever greater insight and through the body to understand our mind and reach our soul. To a yogi, the body is a laboratory for life, a field of experimentation and perpetual research.

For the yogi, the physical body corresponds to one of the elements of nature, namely the earth. We are mortal clay, and we return to dust. All cultures recognize this truth, but nowadays we treat it as a mere metaphor. It is more than that. As you explore your own body, you are in fact exploring this element of nature itself. You are also developing the qualities of earth within yourself: solidity, shape, firmness, and strength.

I have described the yogasanas at length in my earlier books. In this chapter, we will discuss asana not in terms of the techniques of each position but in terms of the qualities and attributes that one must strive for in all asana and in life. As we perfect asana, we will come to understand the true nature of our embodiment, of our being, and of the divinity that animates us. And when we are free from physical disabilities, emotional disturbances, and mental distractions, we open the gates to our soul (*atma*). To understand this, one must gain far more than technical proficiency, and one must do asana not merely as a physical exercise but as a means to understand and then integrate our body with our breath, with our mind, with our intelligence, with our consciousness, with our conscience, and with our core. In this way, one can experience true integration and reach the ultimate freedom.

The True Nature of Health

Most people ask only from their body that it does not trouble them. Most people feel that they are healthy if they are not suffering from illness or pain, not aware of the imbalances that exist in their bodies and minds that ultimately will lead to disease. Yoga has a threefold impact on health. It keeps healthy people healthy, it inhibits the development of diseases, and it aids recovery from ill health.

But diseases are not just a physical phenomenon. Anything that disturbs your spiritual life and practice is a disease and will manifest eventually in illness. Because most modern people have separated their minds from their bodies and their souls have been banished from their ordinary lives, they forget that the well-being of all three (body, mind, and spirit) are intimately entwined like the fibers of our muscles.

Health begins with firmness in body, deepens to emotional stability, then leads to intellectual clarity, wisdom, and finally the unveiling of the soul. Indeed health can be categorized in many ways. There is physical health, which we are all familiar with, but there is also moral health, mental health, intellectual health, and even the health of our consciousness, health of our conscience, and ultimately divine health. These are relative to and depend upon the stage of consciousness we are at, which will be dealt with in chapter 5.

But a yogi never forgets that health must begin with the body. Your body is the child of the soul. You must nourish and train your child.

Physical health is not a commodity to be bargained for. Nor can it be swallowed in the form of drugs and pills. It has to be earned through sweat. It is something that we must build up. You have to create within yourself the experience of beauty, liberation, and infinity. This is health. Healthy plants and trees yield abundant flowers and fruits. Similarly, from a healthy person, smiles and happiness shine forth like the rays of the sun.

The practice of yogasana for the sake of health, to keep fit, or to maintain flexibility is the external practice of yoga. While this is a legitimate place to begin, it is not the end. As one penetrates the inner body more deeply, one's mind becomes immersed in the asana. The first external practice remains dry and peripheral, while the second more intense practice literally soaks the practitioner with sweat, making him wet enough to pursue the deeper effects of the asana.

Do not underestimate the value of asana. Even in simple asanas, one is experiencing the three levels of the quest: the external quest, which brings firmness of the body; the internal quest, which brings steadiness of intelligence; and the innermost quest, which brings benevolence of spirit. While a beginner is not generally aware of these aspects while performing the asana, they are there. Often, we hear people saying that they remain active and light when they do just a little bit of asana practice. When a raw beginner experiences this state of well-being, it is not merely the external or anatomical effects of yoga. It is also about the internal physiological and psychological effects of the practice.

As long as the body is not in perfect health, you are caught in body consciousness alone. This distracts you from healing and culturing the mind. We need sound bodies so we can develop sound minds.

Body will prove to be an obstacle unless we transcend its limitations and remove its compulsions. Hence, we have to learn how to explore beyond our known frontiers, that is to expand and interpenetrate our awareness and how to master ourselves. Asana is ideal for this.

The keys to unlocking our potential are the qualities of purity and sensitivity. The point about purity, or simply cleanliness as it is often called in yoga texts, is not primarily a moral one. It is that purity permits sensitivity. Sensitivity is not weakness or vulnerability. It is clarity of perception and allows judicious, precise action.

On the other hand, rigidity comes from impurity, from accumulated toxins, whether in the physical sense or the mental, when we call it prejudice or narrow-mindedness. Rigidity is insensitivity. The sweat of exertion and the insight of penetration bring us, through a process of elimination and self-cultivation, both purity and sensitivity.

Purity and sensitivity benefit us not only in relation to the inward journey but in relation to our outer environment, the external world. The effects of impurity are highly undesirable. They cause us to develop a hard shell around us. If we construct a stiff shell between ourselves and the world outside our skin, we rob ourselves of most of life's possibilities. We are cut off from the free flow of cosmic energy. It becomes difficult in every sense to let nourishment in or to let toxic waste out. We live in a capsule, what a poet called a "vain citadel."

As mammals, we are homeostatic. That means we maintain certain constant balances within our bodies, temperature for example, by adapting to change and challenge in the environment. Strength and flexibility allow us to keep an inner balance, but man is trying more and more to dominate the environment rather than control himself. Central heating, air conditioning, cars that we take out to drive three hundred yards, towns that stay lit up all night, and food imported from around the world out of season are all examples of how we try to circumvent our duty to adapt to nature and instead force nature to adapt to us. In the process, we become both weak and brittle. Even many of my Indian students who all now sit on chairs in their homes are becoming too stiff to sit in lotus position easily.

Suppose you lose your job. That is an external challenge with attendant worries such as how to pay the mortgage and feed and clothe

the family. It is an emotional upheaval too. But if you are in balance, if there is an energetic osmosis between you and the outer world, you will adapt and survive by finding another job. Purity and sensitivity mean that we receive a cosmic paycheck each day of our lives. When harmony and integration begin through practice in our inner layers of being, there is immediately a beginning to harmony and integration with the world we live in.

A great boon of yoga, even for relative beginners, is the happiness it brings, a state of self-reliant contentment. Happiness is good in itself and a basis for progress. An unquiet mind cannot meditate. A happy and serene mind allows us to pursue our quest as well as live with artistry and skill. Does not the American Declaration of Independence talk of Life, Liberty, and the Pursuit of Happiness? If a yogi had written that, he would have said Life, Happiness, and the Pursuit of Liberty. Sometimes happiness may bring stagnation, but if freedom comes from disciplined happiness, there is the possibility of true liberation.

As I have said, the body should be neither neglected nor pampered, for it is the only instrument and the only resource we are provided with which to embark on the Pursuit of Liberty. At times it is fashionable to despise the body as something non-spiritual. Yet none can afford to neglect it. At other times it is fashionable to indulge the body and to despise what is not physical. Yet none can deny that there is more to life than mere physical pleasure and pain. If we abandon or indulge our bodies, sickness comes, and attachment to it increases. Your body no longer can serve as the vehicle for the inward journey and weighs like a millstone around your neck on the right royal road to the soul. If you say you are your body, you are wrong. If you say you are not your body, you are also wrong. The truth is that although body is born, lives, and dies, you cannot catch a glimpse of the divine except through the body.

Yoga sees the body quite differently than Western sports, which treats the body like a racehorse, trying to push it faster and faster and competing with all other bodies in speed and strength. There are today in India yoga "Olympics" where yoga practitioners can compete with one another. I do not decry this. In my life, I have given many demonstrations around the world in an attempt to popularize yoga. While this was yoga as an exhibition of art, the essence of yoga is not about external display but internal cultivation. Yoga is beautiful as well as Divine. Ultimately, the yogi searches for the inner light as well as inner beauty, infinity, and liberation. Once I was called "Iron Iyengar" by a journalist, and I had to correct him that I am not hard like iron, but hard like a diamond. The hardness of a diamond is part of its usefulness, but its true value is in the light that shines through it.

How then should we approach and practice asana in a way that leads to health and purity? What is the way that leads from flexibility on to divinity? The *Yoga Sutras* by the sage Patanjali provides the foundation for the yogic life. Interestingly it has only four verses that deal specifically with asana. Each mention then is all the more worthy of close reading and deep understanding. Patanjali said that asanas bring perfection in body, beauty in form, grace, strength, compactness, and the hardness and brilliance of a diamond. His basic definition of asana is, "*Sthira sukham asanam.*" *Shtira* means firm, fixed, steadfast, enduring, lasting, serene, calm, and composed. *Sukha* means delight, comfort, alleviation, and bliss. *Asanam* is the Sanskrit plural for asana. The presentation of an asana should therefore be undisturbed, unperturbed, and unruffled at all levels of body, mind, and soul. Or, as I have translated it before, "Asana is perfect firmness of body, steadiness of intelligence, and benevolence of spirit."

Ultimately, when all the sheaths of the body and all the parts of a person coordinate together while performing an asana, you experience the cessation of the fluctuations of the mind and also freedom from afflictions. In asana you must align and harmonize the physical body and all the layers of the subtle emotional, mental, and spiritual body. This is integration. But how does one align these sheathes and experience this integration? How do we find such profound transformation in what from the outside may look simply like stretching or twisting the body into unusual positions? It begins with *awareness*.

Awareness: Every Pore of the Skin Has to Become an Eye

We think of intelligence and perception as taking place exclusively in our brains, but yoga teaches us that awareness and intelligence must permeate the body. Each part of the body literally has to be engulfed by the intelligence. We must create a marriage between the awareness of the body and that of the mind. When the two parties do not cooperate, there is unhappiness on both sides. This leads to a sense of fragmentation and "dis-ease." For example, we should eat only when our mouths spontaneously salivate, as it is the body's intelligence telling us that we are truly hungry. If not, we are force-feeding ourselves and disease will surely follow.

Many moderns use their bodies so little that they lose the sensitivity of this bodily awareness. They move from bed to car to desk to car to couch to bed, but there is no awareness in their movement, no intelligence. There is no action. *Action is movement with intelligence.* The world is filled with movement. What the world needs is more conscious movement, more action. Yoga teaches us how to infuse our movements with intelligence, transforming them into action. In fact action that is introduced in an asana should excite the intelligence, whereas normally the mind gets caught and excited in motion alone. An example of the latter is when you get passionately caught up in watching a football game. That is not yoga. Yoga is when you initiate an action in asana, and somewhere else in the body, something else moves without your permission. The intelligence questions this and asks, "Is that right or wrong? If wrong, what can I do to change it?"

How does one develop this intelligence in the body? How do we learn to turn our movement into action? Asana can begin to teach us. We are developing such an intense sensitivity that each pore of the skin acts as an inner eye. We become sensitive to the interface between skin and flesh. In this way, our awareness is diffused throughout the periphery of our body and is able to sense whether in a particular asana our body is in alignment. You can adjust and balance the body gently from within with the help of these eyes. This is different from seeing with your normal two eyes. Instead you are feeling; you are sensing the position of your body. When you stand in the warrior pose with your arms extended, you can see the fingers of your hand in front of you, but you can also feel them. You can sense their position and their extension right to the tips of your fingers. You can also sense the placement of your back leg and tell whether it is straight or not without looking back or in a mirror. You must observe and correct the body position (adjusting it from both sides) with the help of the trillions of eyes that you have in the form of cells. This is how you begin to bring awareness to your body and fuse the intelligence of brain *and* brawn. This intelligence should exist everywhere in your body and throughout the asana. The moment you lose the feeling in the skin, the asana becomes dull, and the flow or current of the intelligence is lost.

The sensitive awareness of the body and the intelligence of the brain and heart should be in harmony. The brain may instruct the body to do a posture, but the heart has to feel it too. The head is the seat of intelligence; the heart is the seat of emotion. Both have to work in cooperation with the body.

There is an exercise of will, but the brain must be willing to listen to the body and see what is reasonable and prudent within the body's capacity. The intelligence of the body is a fact. It is real. The intelligence of the brain is only imagination. So the imagination has to be made real. The brain may dream of doing a difficult back bend today, but it cannot force the impossible even onto a willing body. We are always trying to progress, but inner cooperation is essential.

Your brain may say, "We can do it." But the knee may say, "Who are you to dictate to me? It is for me to say whether I can do it or not." So you have to listen to what the body says. Sometimes the body cooperates with you, and sometimes it thinks things over. If necessary, use your intelligence to reflect. Solutions will present themselves even though this is initially through trial and error. Then you will have true understanding between the body and the mind, but this requires the humility of the brain and also understanding in the body. The brain does not know everything. If the brain receives knowledge from the body, it will be able to increase the intelligence of the body later. In this way, the body and the brain begin working together to master the asana.

This is the process of interweaving and interpenetration, when the sheaths or layers of being work in harmony with one another. By interweaving, I mean that all the threads and fibers of our being at every level are drawn into contact and communication with each other. This is how the body and the mind learn to work together. The skin provides our outermost layer of intelligence. At our core lies our innermost wisdom. So the knowledge from outer perception and inner wisdom should always be in contact in your postures. At that time there is no duality; you are one; you are complete. You exist without the feeling of existence. The challenge from the skin should tap the Self, our Soul, and the Self has to ask, "What more have I to do?" The external knowledge incites the Self to act.

As I have said, while doing yoga, the body must tell one what to do, not the brain. Brain has to cooperate with the message it receives from the body. I will often say to a student, "Your brain is not in your body! That is why you can't get the asana." I mean of course that his intelligence is in his head and not filling his body. It may be that your brain moves faster than your body or your body may fail to fulfill the instructions of your brain owing to lack of right guidance from your intelligence. You must learn to move the brain a bit more slowly so that it follows the body, or you have to make the body move faster to match the intelligence of the brain. Let the body be the doer, the brain the observer.

After acting, reflect on what you have done. Has the brain interpreted the action correctly? If the brain does not observe correctly, then there is confusion in action. The duty of the brain is to receive knowledge from the body and then guide the body to further refine the action. Pause and reflect between each movement. This is progression in attention. Then in the stillness, you can be filled with awareness. Ask yourself, "Has every part of me done its job?" The Self has to find out whether this has been done well or not.

Pausing to reflect on your movement does not mean that you are not reflecting throughout the movement. There should be constant analysis throughout the action, not just afterward. This leads to true understanding. The real meaning of knowledge is that action and analysis synchronize. Slow motion allows reflective intelligence. It allows our minds to watch the movement and leads to a skillful action. The art of yoga lies in the acuity of observation.

When we ask ourselves, "What am I doing?" and "Why am I doing it?" our minds open. This is self-awareness. However, it is necessary to point out that students should be self-aware, not self-conscious. Self-consciousness is when the mind constantly worries and wonders about itself, doubting and being self-absorbed. It is like having the devil and angel sitting on your shoulders constantly arguing over what you should do. When you are self-conscious, you are going to exhaust yourself. You are also going to strain the muscles unnecessarily because you are thinking about the asana and how far you want to stretch and not experiencing the asana and stretching according to your capacity.

Self-awareness is the opposite of self-consciousness. When you are self-aware, you are fully within yourself, not outside yourself looking in. You are aware of what you are doing without ego or pride.

When you cannot hold the body still, you cannot hold the brain still. If you do not know the silence of the body, you cannot understand the silence of the mind. Action and silence have to go together. If there is action, there must also be silence. If there is silence, there can be conscious action and not just motion. When action and silence combine like the two plates of a car's clutch, it means that intelligence is in gear.

While doing the postures, your mind should be in an interior conscious state that does not mean sleep; it means silence, emptiness, space that can then be filled with an acute awareness of the sensations given by the posture. You watch yourself from inside. It is a full silence. Maintain a detached attitude toward the body and, at the same time, do not neglect any part of the body or show haste but remain alert while doing the asana. Rushing saps the strength, whether you are in Delhi or New York. Do things rhythmically with a calm mind.

It is difficult to speak of bodily knowledge in words. It is much easier to experience it, to discover what it feels like. It is as if the rays of light of your intelligence were shining through your body, out your arms to your fingertips and down your legs and out through the soles of your feet. As this happens, the mind becomes passive and begins to relax. This is an alert passivity and not a dull, empty one. The state of alert repose regenerates the mind and purifies the body.

As you are doing an asana, you have to recharge your intellectual awareness all the time; that means the attention flows without interruption. The moment you collapse, you do not recharge, and the attention is dispersed. Then, the practice of the asana is a habit, not an invigorating creative practice. The moment you bring attention, you are creating something, and creation has life and energy. Awareness allows us to overcome tiredness and exhaustion in our poses and in our lives. For yogis who go out of their way to help those who come to them, fatigue always eats at us. It is an occupational hazard of a yoga teacher. So we have to accept the fatigue and reapply ourselves with intense awareness to regenerate the body and to gain back energy. Awareness in action brings back energy and rejuvenates the body and mind. Awareness brings life. Life is dynamic, and so therefore the asanas should also be.

Dynamic Extension: From the Core of Your Being

The goal of all asana practice is doing them from the core of your being and extending out dynamically through to the periphery of your body. As you stretch, in turn the periphery relates messages back to the core. From head to heels, you must find your center, and from this center you must extend and expand longitudinally and latitudinally. If extension is from the intelligence of the brain, expansion is from the intelligence of the heart. While doing asana, both the intellectual intelligence and the emotional intelligence have to meet and work together. Extension is attention, and expansion is awareness, I often say. It is the bringing of attention and awareness to the tips of your body and activating the skin.

While practicing the asana, it is very important to develop the sensitivity in the skin. One has to create room between the skin and the underlying tissue so that there is no friction between them. The tissues contain the motor nerves, and the skin contains the sensory nerves. They have to function with an understanding of each other in an asana in order to make the intelligence circulate freely without interruption in the body. This is somewhat like an otter that is attached to its skin only through its nose, four paws, and tail and appears to move freely around within.

Extension and expansion always stay firmly rooted in one's center. They originate in the core of one's being. When most people stretch, they simply stretch *to* the point that they are trying to reach, but they forget to extend and expand from where they are. When you extend and expand, you are not only stretching *to*, you are also stretching *from*. Try holding out your arm at your side and stretch it. Did your whole chest move with it? Now try to stay centered and extend out your arm to your fingertips. Did you notice the difference? Did you notice the space that you created and the way in which you stretched from your core? Now try expanding your arm outward in every direction like the circumference of a circle. The stretch should bring the sensitivity and experience of creating space in every direction.

Overstretching occurs when one loses contact with one's center, with the divine core. Instead, the ego wants simply to stretch further, to reach the floor, regardless of its ability, rather than extending gradually from the center. Each movement must be an art. It is an art in which the Self is the only spectator. Keep your attention internal, not external, not worrying about what others see, but what the Self sees. Do not fixate on how far you want to stretch, but in doing the stretch correctly. Do not focus on where you want to go but on going as far as you can with dynamic extension.

One should not overstretch, nor understretch. If one thing is overstretched, something else gets understretched. If overstretching comes from a swollen ego, then understretching results from a lack of confidence. If overstretching is exhibitionism, understretching is escapism. Overstretching and understretching are both wrong: Always stretch from the source, the core, and the foundation of each asana. This is the art of dynamic extension. It is not yoga that injures, but it is the way one does yoga that leads to injury. The moment space becomes narrow, it means you are injuring. In the correct asana, there is no narrowness. Even if your body is stiff, you have to bring space.

Always try to *extend and expand* the body. Extension and expansion bring space, and space brings freedom. Freedom is precision, and precision is divine. From freedom of the body comes freedom of the mind and then the Ultimate Freedom. The Ultimate Freedom that yoga works toward can be tasted in our own bodies, as each limb gains independence, flexibility, and freedom from its neighboring limbs. Certainly, stiffness and rigidity in the body is like wearing a straightjacket or living one's life in a prison.

The movement of the skin gives the understanding of the asana. You must feel the extension to the limits of your skin. As I have said, the skin is the brain of the body, telling what is happening everywhere. The skin, like a mirror, reflects one's mental state, whether tight, slack, flaccid, swollen, tremulous, or stuck. So watch the quality of the skin in practice.

When you extend to your skin, you are also extending your nerve endings. Extending them opens them so that they can throw out their stored impurities. That is why I teach extension and expansion. The nerves release and relax. You feel as if you are extending the skin, the muscles, and even the bones of your body. Practice asanas by creating space in the muscles and skin, so that the body fits into the asana. To do this, the whole body has to act. To extend the part, you must extend the whole.

If the stretch is even, throughout the whole body, there is no strain at all. This does not mean that there is no exertion. There is exertion, but this exertion is exhilaration. There is no wrong stress or strain. A state of elation is felt within. When there is strain, the practice of yoga is purely physical and leads toward imbalances and misjudgment. One feels weary and tired and gets irritated and disturbed. When one stops straining and the brain is passive, it becomes spiritual yoga. When you have extended to the extreme, live in that asana, and experience the joy of freedom in that asana. While stretching, you must always create space and extend from your center. Compression is bondage, and expansion is freedom.

Horizontal expansion and vertical extension should synchronize so that you are extending in all directions. Freedom in a posture is when every joint is active. Let us be full in whatever posture it is we are doing just as we should be full in whatever we do in our lives. In postures it is important to study how far our awareness is extending from the center, how far it penetrates. As the river flows to the sea uninterrupted, our extension should be one single action with single attention. Like the river, your movements should be in that one single action from start to finish. In this way, the energy in our nervous systems flows like the river. As you extend, see whether the energy flows without interruption or not. Everywhere you extend, you are going toward the cosmos. Your energy extends through to the tips of your skin and beyond. This is the secret that martial artists use to generate extraordinary force. They do not punch a brick, they punch through it. Extend the energy of the asana out through your extremities. Let the river flow through you.

Extension is freedom, and freedom allows for relaxation. When there is relaxation in the asana, there is no fatigue. However, you must know the difference between relaxation and laxity. In laxity there is chaos and heedlessness as well as carelessness, and therefore the flow of energy is erratic. In relaxation there is careful adjustment, and hence energy is rhythmic. While in relaxation in the asana, we move outward, and we also remain centered in our core, extending outward and penetrating inward. This is what Patanjali meant when he says in his second *sutra* on asana that "Perfection is achieved when the effort to perform it becomes effortless and the infinite being within is reached."

Relaxation: In Every Pose There Should Be Repose

There is always relaxation in the right position, even though you are fully stretching. The ego is an unrelenting task master. It does not know that one must balance activity and passivity in the asana, exertion and relaxation. When one extends and relaxes, there is no oscillation of mind or body. Balance of activity and passivity transforms the active brain into a witness. This involves keeping the brain passive and the cells of the body active without gripping the muscles. When there is only exertion, one keeps a constant load on the muscles, which tire due to overstretching, and injury occurs. The mind does not balance when you force.

Relaxation means release of unnecessary muscular tension in your body, which also allows firmness of the inner body and serenity in the mind. But how does one experience this peace as one is struggling with the body? How does one experience this serenity as one is feeling the aches and pains of learning the asana? We will return to the subject of pain later and discuss how one can come to see it with equanimity, firmness, and serenity. Here we will give some clues to how to relax in an asana, how to lighten the body, and how to avoid rigidity and hardness.

Begin your asana by releasing the breath till you feel a quiet state of silence in the cells and self. Inhalation is tension, exhalation is freedom. All movements should be done with exhalation. Exhalation purges the stress and tension of the body.

After doing the asana, if you want to stretch deeper, exhale and stretch again. Readjusting the asana after exhalation works on the inner organic body, whereas if done by inhalation it acts on the external physical body. Although a final asana can be judged objectively only from the exterior, it is sustained from within. After reaching the final pose, one has to learn to let go of the effort and tautness of the muscles and shift the load onto the ligaments and joints so that they hold the asana steadily without even the breath causing the body to waver.

Focus on relaxing as you hold the stretch, not clenching, but relaxing and opening. This relaxes the brain as well as the body. You must relax the neck and head as well. If you keep the back skin of the neck passive and the tongue soft, there is no tension in the brain. This is silence in action, relaxation in action. As soon as you learn how to relax the tongue and throat, you know how to relax the brain, because there is also a connection between the tongue and the throat and the brain. The throat, according to yoga, is the region of *vishuddhi chakra*, a purifying wheel. As long as the throat is tense inside, not relaxed, it is an impure wheel. Tightness suggests an intoxication that induces a more general impurity. Look at the Soul, not the Ego. If your throat is tense while doing an asana or pranayama, you are doing it with your egoistic brain instead of your body. Do not clench your teeth or you will also be "clenching" your brain. These are things that you can notice when you are sitting in your office working as well as when you are doing the yogasana practice.

Notice your eyes as well, as you hold the stretch. Tenseness of the eyes also affects the brain. If the eyes are still and silent, the brain is still and passive. The brain can learn only when it begins to relax. When the brain is tense and nervous, chaos sets in, and the brain does not understand anything. The eyes are near the brain, and their behavior reflects the state of the brain. When one is confused, one's brow wrinkles, and the eyes show instability and grow narrow. Compressing the eyes locks the brain and increases stress. When the eyes are wide and open, the brain is eager and receptive. If you are straining the eyes, it means you are living in the world of stress. If the eyes are tense, the brain is doing the asana, not the body. If we look with tension in our eyes, it means our nerves are already exhausted, and we are unnecessarily straining, which causes us to lose energy. In asana practice, we are trying to generate and stabilize our energy, to maintain it and not waste it unnecessarily. Relax the eyes as you look, otherwise you are wasting a great deal of energy.

The eyes should be soft and sunk in. Keep the eyes open and relaxed and at the same time looking backward during your practice. This looking backward educates the eyes to look within and allows you to observe your body and brain. Let your eyes be like flowers, blossoming. Feeling is looking; looking is feeling. You have to feel with your eyes open. If the eyes are outward rather than inward, there is no integration.

When we direct our eyes looking forward from the corner of the temple in its normal field of vision, the frontal brain is working with analysis (*vitarka*). But when we spread our ocular awareness from the back corner of the temple, near the ear, the back brain is brought into play and works with synthesis (*vicara*). The front brain can dismantle because of its powerful penetration. The back brain is holistic and re-assembles. If you find this difficult to imagine, just think what happens when you first walk into a great medieval cathedral. Your eyes may appear to focus on what is before them, the altar for example, but your real awareness takes in the whole immense volume of the space surrounding you, its grandeur and the hum of its ancient silence. This is holistic meditative vision.

While working in asana, if the action is "done" solely from the front brain, it blocks the reflective action of the back brain. The form of each asana needs to be reflected to the wisdom body (*vijnanamaya kosa*) for readjustment and realignment. Whenever asana is done mechanically from the front brain, the action is felt only on the peripheral body, and there is no inner sensation, there is no luminous inner light. If the asana is done with continual reference to the back of the brain, there is a reaction to each action, and there is sensitivity. Then life is not only dynamic, but it is also electrified with life force.

The light and life of our vision should shine everywhere. Finally, the eye of the soul, often called the "third eye," is between your eyebrows but a little higher. If that is still, your soul is still and like a witness observes everything without being affected or enmeshed. So the skin of your brow should be relaxed too.

Relaxation begins from the outer layer of the body and penetrates the deep layers of our existence. Detail and precision of the body lead to mastery of the art of relaxation. One who knows the art of relaxation also knows the art of meditation. Whether one lives in the East or the West, North or South, everyone suffers from stress, and everyone craves rest and relaxation. If one stretches completely, one relaxes completely. Look at a cat, a master of stretching and a master of relaxation. The "effortless effort" that Patanjali describes is also characterized by another important quality, lightness.

Lightness: Think Light and Feel Light

When an asana is done correctly, the body movements are smooth, and there is lightness in the body and freedom in the mind. When an asana is felt as being heavy, it is wrong. You must try to impart a feeling of lightness throughout your body. This can be achieved by mentally extending yourself outward from the center of your body, that is, think tall and act tall. Think not just of raising your arms but of extending them outward in the physical sense, and when you are holding them still, think again of extending the intelligence by reaching still further away from your body. Do not think of yourself as a small, compressed, suffering thing. Think of yourself as graceful and expanding, no matter how unlikely it may seem at the time.

When we lose this lightness, our bodies shrink. The moment the body shrinks, the brain becomes heavy and dull, and you see nothing. The doors of perception are closed. You should immediately lift the intelligence of the chest and open the mind. The corners of the chest are pillars: They should always be firm. Slouching acts like a narcotic to the body. When our parents tell us not to slouch, it is because they instinctively understand that collapsing our chest caves in the very Self. It is because your mind shrinks that your soul shrinks. It is the spine's job to keep the mind alert. To do this, the spine has to keep the brain in position. The spine must never be slack but must reach up to the Self. Otherwise, the divine light within you dims.

As you extend in an asana, you must maintain this lightness. It is for this reason, I say, that in all asanas, ascend to descend and descend to ascend. If we want to touch our toes, for example, we must first stretch upward to open the hinge in the middle of the body, and then we can descend. Similarly, we descend to ascend. We are trying to fill a circle, like in Leonardo DaVinci's famous drawing of human proportions, the Vitruvius Man. We are not trying to break a piece of string by pulling in two different directions. We are seeking the balance of polarity, not the antagonism of duality.

When there is softness in the body and lightness in mind, the asana is correct. Hardness and heaviness mean the asana is wrong. Wherever there is tightness, the brain is overreacting, and you are caught and trapped there; so there is no freedom. Performance from the intellect of the heart, with lightness, firmness, and at the same time softness means it is a total stretch, total extension, and total expansion. Asana done from the brain makes one heavy and done from the heart makes one light.

When should an asana be soft and when should it be rigid? In motion the whole muscle should be like the petals of the flower, open and soft. Never be rigid in motion; only be rigid after you have acquired the position. As a farmer ploughs a field and makes the ground soft, a yogi ploughs his nerves so they can germinate and make a better life. This practice of yoga is to remove weeds from the body so that the garden can grow. If the ground is too hard, what life can grow there? If the body is too stiff and the mind is too rigid, what life can it live?

In contrast to rigidity, tension is not good or bad. It has to be present at the right time in the right amount. Weighing or balancing it evenly is life. There is nothing in this world where yogis say there should be no tension at all. Even dead bodies have tension. You have to find the right amount of tension in your body. The right amount will keep all of your energy in your body. Too much tension is aggression. Injuries come by aggression, by doing aggressive movements, not by doing yoga. But too little tension is weakness. There should be right tension in the body. Right tension is healthy tension. You have to bring everything to life in your body. Remember: Never be rigid in motion. Extension is tension, but it is different than rigidity. Rigidity makes us brittle and causes us to lose our balance. Balance must be achieved at every level of our body and our being.

Balance: Evenness Is Harmony

Through yoga one can begin to develop a perfect balance between both sides of the body. All of us begin with imbalances, favoring one side or the other. When one side is more active than the other, the active side must become the guru for the inactive side to make it equally active. To the weaker side, we must apply attention. We must also show more care. We show keener interest to improve a dull and struggling friend than for an eager and intelligent one. In the same way you have to show yourself this same compassion and act on the weaker side of the body while taking pleasure in the achievement of the active side.

Precision in action comes when the challenge by one side of the body is met by an equal counter-challenge of the other. This ignites the light of knowledge. You must keep your balance by using the intelligence of the body (whether instinct, feeling, or ability) but not by strength. When you keep the balance by strength, it is physical action; when by intelligence of the body, it is relaxation in action. Evenness is harmony, and in that evenness alone you learn.

Seek balance of awareness in all positions by observing the differences on the right and left as well as the intensity of stretch from plane to plane, limb to limb, muscle to muscle, joint to joint, and from bottom to top, side to side, and back to front. Create equal stretch, equal stability, equal spacing, and equal intensity of movement. To bring a part of the body in correct alignment, you have to work with the whole body. You have to work with each and every part of the body. For each asana or pranayama, you have to know what the function or state of each area and each part of the body should be, whether active or passive, stable or mobile. When performing asanas, no part of the body should be idle, no part should be neglected. If you are stretching the right leg, for example, the left leg should not be forgotten. On the contrary you have to alert the left leg to remain stable. This complementary action frees up the right leg to move with ease. Extend where the body is not moving. If you perspire on one side, you should also evenly perspire on the other. When you perspire more on one side, you have not used the other portion fully. Perspiration should be even but not excessive.

In each asana, if the contact between the body and the floor—the foundation—is good, the asana will be performed well. Always watch your base: Be attentive to the portion nearest the ground. Correct first from the root. The standing poses are meant to begin providing this foundation for life. They strengthen the ankles and the knees. When a person is mentally disturbed or dejected, you'll notice he can't stand firmly on his feet. These postures teach one how to stand straight so that the brain can float in its position. Feet are like the root of a tree. If one can't stand properly on one's feet, one develops a negative attitude toward life, and one's yoga too becomes unsteady. These postures help one to maintain stability in times of difficulty and even when catastrophes occur. When stability becomes a habit, maturity and clarity follow. Stability requires balance.

Balance does not mean merely balancing the body. Balance in the body is the foundation for balance in life. In whatever position one is in, or in whatever condition in life one is placed, one must find balance. Balance is the state of the present—the here and now. If you balance in the present, you are living in Eternity. When the intellect is stable, there is no past, no future, only present. Do not live in the future; only the present is real. The mind takes you constantly to the future, as it plans, worries, and wonders. Memory takes you to the past, as it ruminates and regrets. Only the Self takes you to the present, for the divine can be experienced only now. The past, present, and future are held together in each asana as thought, word, and deed become one.

One has to find the median line of each asana so that the energy is properly distributed. When one wavers from the median line, then one goes either to the past or the future. Vertical ascending is the future; vertical descending is the past. The horizontal is the present. The present is the perfect asana. When you open horizontally, future and past meet in the present. This is how dynamic extension and expansion allow you to find balance and live more fully in the present through your body. In asana, we find balance and integration in the three dimensions of space, but we also find balance and integration in the fourth dimension of time.

The ancient sages said that the key to life was balance, balance as I have emphasized in every layer of our being. But what are we supposed to balance? The answer lies in the three qualities of nature, which are called the *guna*. These three qualities must be balanced in your asana practice and in your body, mind, and soul. Roughly they are translated as solidity, dynamism, and luminosity.

We have seen that the essence of nature is change, a never-ending expression and re-expression of itself. What, we must ask ourselves, constantly provokes that change? Why do things simply not stay as they are? This is because of the guna, the three complementary forces that Indian philosophy identifies as emerging from the very root of nature at the moment of creation. Understanding the guna, these three forces of nature, will be important for the success of your practice of yogasana and your inward journey to the Universal Soul.

As soon as nature becomes manifest, these three forces shift. They lose their balance and create instability. That instability is very fertile. Mathematicians say that numbers progress from one to two to three to many. It is the number three that unlocks the possibility of infinite diversity. Infinite, unmanifested origin is one. Duality is two. Duality is the idea or concept of separation, of division, but alone it cannot manifest in phenomena. Three is a wave, a sine curve, a vibration like light or sound. When two waves collide, a new phenomenon is created. That is the creativity inherent in nature. Even at the subtlest level, that of vibration and infra-atomic particles, nature's built-in wobble sets it on an endless cycle of creation, destruction, and recreation. From three comes many.

As I said, the guna is made up of three complementary forces. They are: *tamas* (mass or inertia), *rajas* (vibrancy or dynamism), and *sattva* (luminosity or the quality of light).

Let us look at a practical example. In asana, we are trying to broach the mass of our gross body, to break up the molecules and divide them into atoms that will allow our vision to penetrate within. Our body resists us. It is mulish. It will not budge. Why? Because in body tamas predominates. It has to. Body needs mass, bones need density, and sinew and muscle need solidity and firmness. To be firm-fleshed is desirable; to be slack-muscled is not.

Density in bones is a virtue, but in brains it is a vice. You hear people say, "He's thick," or "Don't be dense," because in our brain and nervous system, rajas (dynamism and vibrancy) should predominate, and density is a liability. Whereas mind is naturally quick, mercurial, and slippery, body tends to heaviness, inertia, and sluggishness. An excess is unwelcome; a muscle-bound body is like a very heavy car with a small engine; it will only move slowly. More than that, it takes more energy to overcome inertia than to pick up speed. For example, it is more difficult to push a stationary car up to one mile per hour than to push it from one mile per hour to two miles per hour.

With regard to asana practice, this means that initially we need to exert ourselves more as resistance is greater. Of the two aspects of asana, exertion of our body and penetration of our mind, the latter is eventually more important. Penetration of our mind is our goal, but in the beginning to set things in motion, there is no substitute for sweat.

But once there is movement and then momentum, penetration can start. When effort becomes effortless, asana is at its highest level. Inevitably this is a slow process, and if we break off our practice, inertia reasserts itself. What we are really doing is infusing dense matter with vibrant energy. That is why good practice brings a feeling of lightness and vitality. Though the mass of our body is heavy, we are meant to tread lightly on this earth.

We must be clear that the key issue is one of appropriate proportion and balance in the guna according to the material phenomenon involved. For example, it is appropriate for a table to be very *tamasic*. If we want it to be more *rajasic*, we add wheels and call it a trolley. Tamas gives density and mass, and when these qualities exceed our needs, we call it dullness and inertia. An inert mass is one that we cannot energize with rajas.

The negative aspect of rajas is turbulent, frenetic, and agitated. We want a quick mind, not an agitated one. We also want a calm, clear mind, which brings us to sattva. These words express a value, rather than an explicit reality. The truth is that we experience too little of sattva to know it well. The solidity of tamas and the eye-drawing movement of rajas eclipse our view. In a world of objects and sensory excitement, tamas and rajas reign. But if you can come to yoga with a wish to learn how truly to relax and yet remain alert, you are really saying that you would like sattva to play a more prominent role in your life. We use the word luminosity, which is the inner, serene quality of light, to describe sattva. It is that quality we are trying to elevate and integrate within us. Luminosity is clear, alert, and tranquil.

The interplay of these three guna forces is of crucial importance in your yoga practice. You have to learn to identify and observe them in order to be able to adjust and balance their proportions and as you penetrate inward, bring the beauty of sattva to the surface. You are like an artist with three basic pigments on his palette, forever remixing and blending them in order to express the right combination of color, form, and light on your canvas. It is through the ability to do this that you can also avoid pain and heal diseases whether they are at mental, emotional, or physical stages of manifestation. Since pain is an unavoidable part of asana practice, it must now be addressed in its own right.

Pain: Find Comfort Even in Discomfort

Many people focus on the past or the future to avoid experiencing the present, often because the present is painful or difficult to endure. In yoga class, many students think that they must simply "grit their teeth and bear it" until the teacher tells them they can come out of the asana. This is seeing yoga as calisthenics and is the wrong attitude. The pain is there as a teacher, because life is filled with pain. In the struggle alone, there is knowledge. Only when there is pain will you see the light. Pain is your guru. As we experience pleasures happily, we must also learn not to lose our happiness when pain comes. As we see good in pleasure, we should learn to see good in pain. Learn to find comfort even in discomfort. We must not try to run from the pain but to move through and beyond it. This is the cultivation of tenacity and perseverance, which is a spiritual attitude toward yoga. This is also the spiritual attitude toward life.

Just as the ethical codes of yoga purify our actions in the world, the asanas and pranayama purify our inner world. We use these practices to help us learn to bear and overcome the inevitable pains and afflictions of life. Let me give you an example. To detect diabetes, one takes a test to see how well sugar is tolerated in the body. Similarly the practices of yoga show us how much pain the body can bear and how much affliction the mind can tolerate. Since pain is inevitable, asana is a laboratory in which we discover how to tolerate the pain that cannot be avoided and how to transform the pain that can. While we do not actively seek out pain, we do not run from the inevitable pain that is part of all growth and change. The asanas help us to develop greater tolerance in body and mind so that we can bear the stress and strain more easily. In other words, the effort and its unavoidable pains are an essential part of what the asanas can teach us. Back bends, for example, allow us to see the courage and tenacity of people, to see whether they can bear the pain. Balancing asanas on the arms teach and cultivate tolerance. If you can adapt to and balance in a world that is always moving and unstable, you learn how to become tolerant to the permanence of change and difference.

Endurance is needed to remain in an asana. To master an asana, you need patience and discipline. The asana will not come by making faces. So how does one learn to make pain bearable? We have already seen how one must create repose in the pose; one must create relaxation even as there is the right amount of tension. This relaxation can start by releasing the stress residing in the temples and in the cells of the brain. This de-stresses the load of the brain, by releasing the eyes and the temples. This in turn takes the stress load off the nerves and muscle fiber. That is how you can convert an unbearable pain into a bearable one, which allows you the time and space in which to eventually master the asana and eradicate the pain all together.

To get freedom, you have to bear the pain. This is equally true in life. My student said that while sitting for pranayama, she got pins and needles in her feet, and all her concentration was on her feet. I told her that what she had done was also good practice. Because it was not serene, she thought she had done it badly. But practice is not just about pleasurable sensations. It is about awareness, and awareness leads us to notice and understand both the pleasure and the pain.

In the beginning, pain can be very strong because the body resists us. By surrendering to it, we soften the body, and gradually it will lessen. But if once we are more proficient and pain returns acutely at a time when it should not be there, it is prudent to leave the asana for a while and reflect on what is going wrong. Pain comes only when the body does not understand how to do the asana, which is the case in the beginning. In the correct posture, pain does not come. To learn the right posture, you have to face the pain. There is no other way.

Your intelligence should have an intimacy with your body. It should be in close contact and know it well. When there is no intimacy between your mind and your body, there is duality, there is separation, and there is no integration. When you experience pain, you come in close contact with the part that is painful, so that you can adjust it and lessen the pain and feel the lightness. Pain is a great philosopher, because it thinks constantly of how to get rid of itself and demands discipline. The other side of the equation of pain is the understanding of how pain brings focus of attention on the affected area. If we release the tension of the brain, that attention shows the way to lessen and later eradicate the source of pain. In this way, pain can be a great teacher, which educates us how to live with it and eventually say goodbye.

It is not just that yoga is causing all of this pain; the pain is already there. It is hidden. We just live with it or have learned not to be aware of it. It is as if your body is in a coma. When you begin yoga, the unrecognized pains come to the surface. When we are able to use our intelligence to purify our bodies, then the hidden pains are dispersed. As long as there is tightness in body and mind, there is no peace. Internal mistakes such as forcing, acting without observing, tightening the throat, and blocking the ears create habits, and these habits create lack of awareness, constriction, heaviness, tightness, imbalance, and pain. For example, when muscles that have atrophied return to life, there are the pangs of rebirth. There are only two ways to confront pain: to live with the pain forever or to work with the pain and see if you can eradicate it.

While we must recognize the existence and importance of pain, we must not glorify it. Where pain exists, there must be a reason for it.

The goal is not to hold at any cost an asana that is painful or to try to achieve it prematurely. This is how I hurt myself as a young practitioner when my teacher demanded that I do the Hanuman asana, which involves an extreme leg stretch, without proper training or preparation. The goal is to do the asana with as much possible intensity of intelligence and love. To do this, one must learn the difference between "right" pain and "wrong" pain.

Right pain is not only constructive but also exhilarating and involves challenge, while wrong pain is destructive and causes excruciating suffering. Right pain is for our growth and for our physical and spiritual transformation. Right pain is usually felt as a gradual lengthening and strengthening feeling and must be differentiated from wrong pain, which is often a sharp and sudden cautionary feeling that our body uses to tell us we have gone too far beyond our present abilities. In addition, if you get a pain that is persistent, and intensifying as you work, it's likely a wrong pain.

The challenge of yoga is to go beyond our limits—*within reason.* We continually expand the frame of the mind by using the canvas of the body. It is as if you were to stretch a canvas more and create a larger surface for a painting. But we must respect the present form of our body. If we pull too fast or too much at once, we will rip the canvas. If the practice of today damages the practice of tomorrow, it is not correct practice.

Many yoga teachers ask you to do the asanas with ease and comfort and without any stress or true exertion. This ultimately leaves the practitioner living within the limits of his or her mind, with the inevitable fear, attachment, and pettiness. These teachers and their students feel that the kind of precise and intense practice I am describing is painful. Yes, it is true that sometimes we experience pain during our practice as we exert ourselves and our will. Yoga is meant for the purification of body and its exploration as well as for the refinement of the mind. This demands strength of will both to observe and at the same time to bear the physical pain without aggravating it. Without certain stress, the true asana is not experienced, and the mind will remain in its limitations and will not move beyond its existing frontiers. This limited state of mind can be described as the petty, small mind.

I remember two students who were top ballet dancers. They could achieve every position without encountering resistance or stress, so the journey to the final posture could teach them nothing. It was my job to take them back into the positions and show them how to create mobility with resistance in themselves so that they could work at the point of balance between the known and unknown. When we extend and expand our body consciousness beyond its present limitations, we are working on the frontier of the known toward the unknown by an intelligent expansion of our awareness. Ballet dancers have the opposite problem to most people in that, because of their excessive flexibility, their physical capacity outstrips their intellectual consciousness.

When we start practicing asanas, we experience both physical and mental pain. Just as we must learn to detect the difference between right physical pain and wrong physical pain, we must do the same with mental pain. Right mental pain should also be gradual and allow us to strengthen and not to snap. Getting up at six in the morning to do yoga before you go to work may seem painful, but it is constructive and involves challenging yourself to go beyond your present limits. However, we must remember to keep our practice progressive and gradual. If you try to get up so early that this pain will cause your body to rebel, say four in the morning, you will not be able to sustain the practice. In addition, if getting up at four in the morning causes you to be short of sleep and irritable with your family, you are being selfish and in addition are transferring your suffering to others. We use right pain like a vaccine against the unavoidable pain and suffering that life always sends our way, but the dose must be correct. Asana practice is an opportunity to look at obstacles in practice and life and discover how we can cope with them.

Many intellectually developed people are still emotionally immature. If they have to face pains, they try to escape from them. They are seldom prepared to face that pain and to work through it when they are taken intensely into a posture. This practice brings them face to face with the reality of their bodies' natures. We must face up to our emotions, not run away from them. We do not do yoga just for enjoyment; we do it for ultimate emancipation.

Most people want to take joy without suffering. I will take both. See how far suffering takes me. When you do not resist suffering, you will make friends with other people who suffer. I suffered a lot in my own body. Now when someone tells me of his sufferings, I feel in my body what that suffering is. My personal experience provides me with great love and compassion. So I say, "My friend, let me try and do something." Pain comes to guide you. When you have known pain, you will be compassionate. Shared joys cannot teach us this.

However, compassion does not mean pity. A surgeon operates on patients, which would be painful for the patients if they were not anaesthetized. As a yoga teacher, I have to operate when the patient is conscious. Obviously it is painful. But it is only in this way that we learn to act, to live, to grow. We all have presence of mind when everything goes well, but we need to have presence of mind when something goes wrong. If we face suffering and accept it as a necessary means, all anxiousness disappears.

Every illness is in reality a part of ourselves; it is a part of our manifestation. According to yogic philosophy, diseases and suffering are the fruits of our past actions. In that sense we are responsible for what we have created. If we confront affliction through yoga, we awaken a new awareness of tolerance and endurance, as well as a true sympathy for others in their afflictions. These qualities indicate the degree of development we have reached. So why not take adversity positively? Certainly it is an alarm signal, but it also contains the seed for its own resolution and transcendence.

In my life I count among my greatest blessings my early ill health, poverty, lack of education, and the harshness of my guru. Without these deprivations, I might never have held on so faithfully to yoga. When everything else is stripped away, the essential is revealed.

Of course, when you are young, it is particularly difficult to know what to hold on to and to have the determination and perseverance to do so. As a struggling youth in Pune, I clung to my yoga practice. As I have said, society as a whole thought anyone who wanted to make a career as a yoga teacher was mad as well as a good for nothing. The climate of opinion was that it was acceptable to become a priest or a renunciate, but yoga as a profession was beyond the pale. An even greater source of pain was my family's disapproval and ostracism. For example, coming from an ultra-orthodox background, I naturally had a *shendi*, the long tuft or lock of hair from the crown of the shaven head. In modern, westernized Pune, this was utterly scorned. My class of college students, all so strong and fit and bright, teased and ridiculed me mercilessly. Eventually I shaved my shendi off and adopted a modern haircut. This brought the wrath of my family down on me. They would not eat with me or allow me in their kitchens.

Hindus are also traditionally forbidden to cross the sea. After my first teaching trip to England in 1954, I stopped in Bangalore to pay my respects to my maternal uncle. He refused to even let me in the house. Is it any wonder I developed a defensive shield of haughtiness as a young man? Time has mellowed me, but in my youth haughtiness was the only way I knew to preserve myself in what seemed a hostile world. Yet this hostility also motivated me to become enduringly faithful to yoga.

Everyone sometimes finds themselves in the awful dilemma when every course of action or behavior seems to be wrong. Arjuna, in chapter 2 of the Bhagavad Gita is on the horns of such a dilemma. To do nothing is an action too, with inevitable consequences, and so that is not a way to escape pain and suffering either. With Krishna's help,

Arjuna follows the path of *dharma,* of the science of religious duty, and so reconciles what is on the human and material level, irreconcilable. In my own youth, it seemed impossible to be accepted by my students and by my family. But by persevering on the yogic path, I attained a level at which I am not only accepted but even now honored by my students and my family. This would have been impossible without the evolution that yoga provided.

In one instance, my trouble quickly turned into a great blessing. Because I was teaching so many women's and girls' classes, it was generally assumed I was guilty of immorality. I even had a row with my guru over this painfully false accusation. But it made me decide to marry even though I was in no financial position to do so, and I should say that my marriage to Ramamani *was* my greatest blessing. So it is by facing up to adversity and suffering, and accepting it as a necessary means, that our anxieties are resolved and disappear. If we are loyal to the path we are on, our lives will get better, and the light of distant perfection will come to illuminate our journeys.

Perfecting: Always Be Happy with the Smallest Improvement

Let the goal be to reach Perfection, but be content with a little progress toward perfection every day. Overambition can be destructive of sustainable progress. Perfection is ultimately only with God. So what is the value of perfection if it can be found only in God? We are creatures who can dream of perfection, and it is this dream that inspires one to improve. It is this dream that ignites the effort needed to transform. Perfection creates interest in art and life. The instinct that draws us toward the dream of perfection is really a desire for God.

Sometimes our body is willing, but our mind is weak and says, "We don't have time," or "Forget it, it's not worth all the effort." Sometimes it is our mind that is willing, but our body is weak and says,

"I'm really too tired for all this trouble." A practitioner must focus between the mind and the body, listening to the counsel of each, but letting the intelligence and the soul make the true decision, for this is where real willpower and real dedication are found. Do to your capacity while always striving to extend your capacity. Ten minutes today. After a few days, twelve minutes. Master that, then again extend. It is better to do a good pose minimum than a bad pose maximum.

Do not say that you are disappointed with yourself. Find time every day to do something to maintain the asana practice. Sometimes both body and mind yield to willpower, and at other times they rebel. Do you have a problem part that makes the practice difficult for you? An injured knee? A stiff back? That is your problem child. Learn how to deal with it and how to nurture it, as you would a child who had problems that needed extra love and attention. Do not bother about failures either. Failures in life lead one toward determination and in having the necessary philosophical approach. Be detached. Look at me, I am not afraid, and I know there is no way to spare my difficulties. For me if it came yesterday, so much the better. If it comes after 20 years, it is also good. All is well.

Do not be afraid. Do not be attached to your body. Even if fear comes, accept it and find the courage to come through it. When you experience fear, you must practice without attachment to the body, thinking of it objectively as an opportunity for creative work. When fear is not there, you can treat the body more subjectively, as a part of yourself that nonetheless requires practice and cultivation.

Long uninterrupted practice of asanas and pranayama, done with awareness, makes the foundation firm and brings success. The young, the old, the extremely aged, even the sick and the infirm obtain perfection in yoga by constant practice. Success will come to the person who practices. Success in yoga is not obtained by the mere reading of sacred texts. These are increasingly essential aids but without practice remain simply theoretical. The test of a philosophy is whether it is applicable and even more so applicable now in how you live your life. Even Patanjali, who was born a spiritual genius, said that yoga is mastered only by long persistent nonstop practice, with zeal and determination.

When the gardener plants an apple seed, does he expect the apples to appear at once? Of course not. The gardener waters the seed, watches each day, and feels happy seeing the growth. Treat the body in the same way. We water our asana and pranayama practice with love and joy seeing the small progress. While we know what the goal is, we do not focus on enlightenment. We know that when our practice is ripe, illumination comes. Patience allied with disciplined practices brings the required willpower.

Willpower is concrete, not ethereal. When you do something, you demonstrate your willpower, and it becomes all the easier to have the same power of will the next time. When you perform your asana, you are physically demonstrating willpower through the expression of the muscles. Willpower is not just in the mind, but it is also in the body. I have been known to slap a man's thigh and say, "Willpower is here." With willpower, you elongate the muscles and bring elegance. This willpower allows us to express peace, contentment, and freedom from body attachment as we expand our minds. Willpower is nothing but willingness to do.

You have to ask yourself, using your intelligence and your willpower, can I do a little better than I am doing? Light comes to a person who extends his awareness a little more than seems possible. We limit ourselves by settling. We say, "Oh, I do not want to go beyond this, because I know this is good." This is living in one's old mind. Question whether you can do a little more. Then immediately you experience that the movement is coming. If you are conscientious, your conscience whispers, "Try to go a little further." If one keeps one's aim to the maximum, Self-knowing will come. I say this because your mind and intelligence move deeper toward the inner body, bringing the mind closer to the Self—the core of being. The moment one goes a little more than the body wants to take, one is nearer the Self. The minute one says, "I am satisfied," the light of awareness and attention is fading.

The role of memory in asana practice is to allow us to compare yesterday's practice with today's so we can see if we are progressing in the right direction. But many people repeat what they have learned in the past, and their presentation of asanas becomes mechanical, which causes the body and mind to stagnate. An asana is not a posture that can ever be assumed mechanically. It involves thought and therefore innovation and improvisation, at the end of which a balance is achieved between movement and resistance. Never repeat: A repetition makes the mind dull. You must always animate and create interest in what you are doing. To illustrate my point, I will sometimes assume a standing asana in front of the class, and I will tell them that what I have done is a perfect asana. Nobody can tell me it has any defect. It is perfect in appearance but dead inside; my mind is elsewhere. Then I redo the asana with my mind fully present. I create unity within me, and I make them see the attention of the legs, torso, and senses of perception. They are perceptively different.

Do not allow past experiences to be imprinted on your mind. Perform asanas each time with a fresh mind and with a fresh approach. If you are repeating what you did before, you are living in the memory, so you are living in the past. That means you don't want to proceed beyond the experience of the past. Retaining that memory is saying, "Yesterday I did it like that." When I ask, "Is there anything new from what I did yesterday?" then there is progress. Am I going forward or am I going backward? Then you understand how to create dynamism in a static asana. That memory has to be used as a springboard from which you can ask yourself, "What more can I do than what I did yesterday?" This is equally true in life as in asana practice. Usually when a person has mastered an asana, it becomes uninteresting. That is why you can see many people mechanically doing the same thing over and over again, but their minds are elsewhere. Blind spots develop, and you cannot savor the asana. It is not the right approach. People think they have attained the end. How can they know? It may be only a beginning. You must always see if you can cross the line of past experiences. You have to create within yourself the feeling of beauty, liberation, and infinity. These can be experienced only in the present.

As we grow more adept and asanas come to us, it becomes tempting to contain our practice within a zone of proficient complacency. I call this "*bhoga* yoga," or yoga exclusively for pleasure. No longer do we employ the mirror of reflexive intelligence to seek out and correct imperfection; we use it for the purpose of self-regarding vanity. The yogic journey is becalmed in the doldrums. If there is no wind in our sails, the only way out is to row. This means to reapply ourselves to zealous, effortful, sustained practice, to lay down a new challenge. What is wrong? Where and how can I improve? This is where the fire of practice (*tapas*) ignites the lamp of intelligence, and self-knowledge (*svadhyaya*) dawns. The word tapas contains the meaning of inner intellectual heat, which burns out our impurities.

If we ever find ourselves apart from or superior to others, purer or more elevated by yoga, we can be sure that we are becalmed or even drifting back into a state of ignorance. It was Ramanuja, the saint and philosopher, who, more than nine hundred years ago, exposed the Brahminical misconception that we can be "above" others. On the contrary, practice and purity of life place us "among" not above. Just as we have discussed inner integration within our own bodies, this naturally leads to integration with all other life. Integrity means one. One is the number that can go into all other numbers. The fully sensitive and sensible being becomes not a "somebody" but the common denominator of humanity. This takes place only when the intelligence of the head is transformed by humility and the wisdom of the heart and compassion is kindled.

If there is an end, then there is no God. Creation by God never ends, so creation of your movements never ceases. The moment you say, "I have got it," you have lost everything you had. As soon as something comes, you have to go one step further. Then there is evolution. The moment you say, "I am satisfied with that," that means stagnation has come. That is the end of your learning; you have closed the windows of your intellect. So let me do what I cannot do, not what I can do. You have always to do a little bit more than you think you can, in quality and in quantity. This is what leads ultimately to beauty and greatness.

As you take great pains to learn, continue with devotion in what you have learned. Learning is very difficult, but it is twice as difficult to keep the ground gained. Soldiers say that it is easier to win a battle than to occupy the territory conquered. While I continually try to improve my practice, I do my best and am contented with what I am able to attain. Even as the body ages and is able to do less, there are subtleties that reveal themselves, which would be invisible to younger or more athletic bodies. You have to create love and affection for your body, for what it can do for you. Love must be incarnated in the smallest pore of the skin, the smallest cell of the body, to make them intelligent so they can collaborate with all the other ones, in the big republic of the body.

This love must radiate from you to others. Practitioners of the asanas alone often forget that yoga is for cultivating the head and heart. Patanjali talked about friendliness, compassion, gladness, and joy. Friendliness and grace are two qualities that are essential for the yoga student. In yoga class, students often look so serious and so separate from one another. Where is the friendliness? Where is the compassion? Where is the gladness? Where is the joy? Without these, we have not achieved the true yoga of Patanjali.

You must purge yourself before finding faults in others. When you see a mistake in somebody else, try to find if you are making the same mistake. This is the way to take judgment and to turn it into improvement. Do not look at others' bodies with envy or with superiority. All people are born with different constitutions. Never compare with others. Each one's capacities are a function of his or her internal strength. Know your capacities and continually improve upon them.

Over time the intensity with which one can practice develops. Yoga identifies four levels of intensity of practice, which relate to the twin aspects of exertion and penetration. Exertion, or our effort through practice, generates the energy, which we need for the journey to penetrate to the core of our being. The first level of intensity is one we all know in which we exert ourselves only a little, perhaps do one class a week and find reasons not to practice at home. We all have to begin yoga somewhere. Mild practice is not bad practice, and it is better to sustain what we can do than to collapse and give up. Naturally this mild investment does not pay big dividends, and in relation to penetration our awareness remains rudimentary and peripheral. We will know, for example, that we can touch our ankles and not our toes.

If we increase our application and devote more time and effort, we will be able to consider ourselves decent average practitioners, not always consistent, but nevertheless the inner structure of our body and organs will begin to reveal itself. We will feel fiber and sinew, liver stretch (as in back bends), and heart's repose.

The next stage is determined and intense. Our inward gaze becomes refined, insightful, judicious, and discerning. We will become aware of our thoughts flickering and how the movement of breath ruffles or calms the consciousness. Our intelligence will awaken to the point where it can see things in their true light and make a myriad of meaningful choices both in life and practice.

The highest level is characterized as relentless, inexorable, a total investment of oneself in practice. It is almost unknown for anyone to be able to plunge into this level from the beginning. Probably the circumstances of life would not allow it initially, but over time it can be reached. Our insight can now finally penetrate through all the tortuous subtleties of cunning ego, our wisdom matures, and we touch the core of being.

The point of such a scale or ladder of intensity is not to make us feel inadequate but for reference purposes, so that we can truly and honestly see where we are and how we are doing. It is analogous to the Biblical parable of the talents of silver that a lord distributed to his servants. Those who fully invested them energetically and wisely were able to return the silver to their lord tenfold and were duly honored. The servant who merely hid his silver away in the ground was able to do no more than return what he had received. His lord was displeased. We all receive God-given talents, and it is our duty to develop them energetically to realize their full potential, otherwise it is as if we are turning our nose up at the gifts of life. But more than that, our talents, however much they may vary from individual to individual, when realized to the full, provide the link that will take us back to a reunion with the divine.

Divine Yoga: Do the Asana with Your Soul

In asana and pranayama practice, we should have the impression we are working on the outer to get closer to the inner reality of our existence. This is true. We work from the periphery to the core. The material body has a practical reality that is accessible. It is here and now, and we can do something with it. However, we must not forget that the innermost part of our being is also trying to help us. It wants to come out to the surface and express itself.

In the example of triangle pose (*Trikonasana*), we notice that, because of the relationship of the posture with our anatomy, we all fall into the same traps. Our body seems to be trying to collapse forward to the floor. Our body does not want to open itself in the way we see in a perfectly expressed asana. So we apply ourselves and learn the adjustments that will cause the whole body to open. We extend and redress our arm, lengthen the chest, and open the pelvis. But we also, in the process of applied learning, open our mind and intelligence. An opening is like a doorway, and there is no such thing as a doorway that you can only go through one way. Yes, we are trying to penetrate in, but what is trying to come out to meet us? It is the light of the innermost sheath of bliss (*ananda*), which wants to shine out. Normally we are like a shuttered lantern; our light within invisible. As we create opening, this draws back the shutter, and the light of the lamp shines out.

In this regard, we should also consider how the heart of nature (*prakrti*) is also willing to help us. The very life force of nature is an initiating power (*prerana*), a driving force, an incitement to creation. It hears our call and responds to it in proportion to the valor and determined intent with which it is invoked. It responds to the exercise of our willpower, so that an intense aspirant will receive higher benefits than a mild one. There is a saying that "God helps those who help themselves." This is also true of nature.

When you do the asana correctly, the Self opens by itself; this is divine yoga. Here the Self is doing the asana, not the body or brain. The Self involves each and every pore of the skin. It is when the rivers of the mind and the body get submerged in the sea of the core that the spiritual discipline commences. There is no special spiritual discipline. When there is passivity, pensiveness, and tranquility of body and mind, do not stick there, but proceed. Here the spiritual experience in yoga commences. No doubt, one may say reading holy books is spiritual practice. But what I teach is spiritual practice in action. As I said at the beginning of this chapter, I use the body to discipline the mind and to reach the soul. Asanas, when done with the right intention, will help to transform an individual by taking the person away from an awareness of just the body toward the consciousness of the soul. Indeed, as I often say, body is the bow, asana the arrow, and soul is the target.

An asana must be righteous and virtuous. By righteous I mean that it must be true. You must not cheat or pretend. You must fill every inch of your body with the asana from your chest and arms and legs to the tips of your fingers and toes so that the asana radiates from the core of your body and fills the entire diameter and circumference of your limbs. You must feel your intelligence, your awareness, and your consciousness in every inch of your body.

By virtuous I mean that it must be done with the right intention, not for ego or to impress but for the Self and to move closer to God. In this way the asana is a sacred offering. We are surrendering our egos. This is supreme devotion to God (*Isvara pranidhana*).

It must not be just your mind or even your body that is doing the asana. You must be in it. You must do the asana with your soul. How can you do an asana with your soul? We can only do it with the organ of the body that is closest to the soul—the heart. So a virtuous asana is done from the heart and not from the head. Then you are not just doing it, but you are in it. Many people try to think their way into an asana, but you must instead feel your way into it through love and devotion.

In this way, you will work from your heart, not your brain, to create harmony. The serenity in the body is the sign of spiritual tranquility. As long as you do not feel the serenity in the body, in each and every joint, there is no chance for emancipation. You are in bondage. So while you are sweating and aching, let your heart be light and let it fill your body with gladness. You are not only becoming free, but you are also being free. What is not to be glad about? The pain is temporary. The freedom is permanent.

In the next chapter, we proceed deeper from the body to the breath, from flesh to vital energy. We will learn more about the role of our energy and of our breath in the next stage of the Inward Journey.

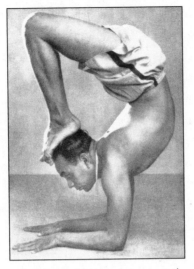

Chapter 3

VITALITY
The Energy Body (*Prana*)

Everyone desires more life energy. If energy could be packaged and sold in a shop, it would be the most successful business ever. Merely talking about energy excites and energizes people. Where can we get it, people want to know. Well, not in packets and not in shops because it is, first, everywhere and, second, free of charge.

We give many names to God, even though He is One. The same is true of energy. There is nuclear energy, electrical energy, muscular energy, and mental energy. All of these are vital energy or life energy, called in Sanskrit, *pranic* energy or simply *prana*. Prana is called Chi in China and Ki in Japan. Some suggest that the nearest traditional concept of prana in the West is the Holy Spirit of Christianity, a sacred power that is both immanent and transcendent. Prana is also often called wind, vital air. The Bible begins its description of Creation with the sentence, "God's breath moved upon the waters." Prana is God's breath. Prana is the energy permeating the universe at all levels. It is physical, mental, intellectual, sexual, spiritual, and cosmic energy.

All vibrating energies are prana. All physical energies such as heat, light, gravity, magnetism, and electricity are also prana. It is the hidden and potential energy in all beings, released to the fullest extent as a response to any threat to one's survival. It is the prime mover of all activity. It is energy that creates, protects, and destroys. Hindus often say that GOD is Generator, Organizer, and Destroyer. Inhalation is the generating power, retention is the organizing power, and exhalation, if the energy is vicious, is the destroyer. This is prana at work. Vigor, power, vitality, life, and spirit are all forms of prana.

Prana is usually translated as breath, yet this is only one of its manifestations. According to the Upanishads, it is the principle of life and consciousness. It is equated with the Soul (*Atman*). It is the breath of life of all beings in the universe. They are born through it and live by it, and when they die their individual breath dissolves into the cosmic breath. It is the most essential, real, and present feature of every moment of our lives and yet it remains the most mysterious. It is yoga's job, and especially *pranayama*'s, to enter into the heart of this mystery.

Prana, in the form of breath, is the starting point. The suffix, *ayama*, means stretch, extension, expansion, length, breadth, regulation, prolongation, restraint, and control. Put in its simplest form, therefore, pranayama means the prolongation and restraint of breath. Since prana is energy and life force, pranayama means the extension and expansion of all our vital energy. It has to be clear that you cannot just increase the volume of anything as volatile and explosive as pure energy without taking steps to contain, harness, and direct it. If you were suddenly to triple the strength of the electrical current arriving in your house, you would not think the kettle would boil in a third of the usual time and your lights burn three times brighter. You know you would immediately burn out all the circuits and be left with nothing. Why should our body be different? That is why Patanjali clearly stated that between the practice of asana and pranayama, there is a step up. There has to exist, through proficiency in asana, strength and stability in the circuitry of the body to withstand the increase in current that pranayama practice will bring.

Many people have approached me over the years full of the woes that befell them because they did not respect this elementary precaution. Often they were ignorant about the need to build a solid foundation and had signed up for various courses in the hope of leaping into a facile spirituality. Their weakness of body and mind betrayed them and compounded their troubles. Patanjali himself warned that if the base is not firm, sorrow, despair, unsteadiness of body, and shakiness of breath will result. Mental depression and accompanying tremors are a serious matter. They are extreme, and in his third *sutra* on asana, Patanjali specifically said that asana practice will protect us from the dangers and vicissitudes of extremes. He called extremes dualities. In this context it means we have to build up sufficient fortitude in body and mind to control ourselves sensibly. To gorge one day and fast the next is not sensible. If an unkind word at the office plunges you into gloom, anger, or resentment, it is not sensible. If we still ricochet between behavioral, emotional, and mental extremes, we are not ready for pranayama. If we have a reasonable strength of body and nerves and stability of emotions and mind, then we are.

For the Inward Journey, we will need a lot of energy, and a very subtle, high-quality energy too. This never-ending exploration, occupation, and illumination requires the special energy of prana. Prana is special because it carries awareness. It is the vehicle of consciousness. If you want to send your awareness to the furthermost cell of your big toe, prana will carry it there. When you have a sufficient flow of prana, you can spread your consciousness everywhere within. To do this you need to generate a lot of prana. To generate prana you must cultivate the extension, expansion, control, and restraint of your normal breath. Just as in the last chapter we were using these same terms about our practice on the physical and outermost sheath of being, the *annamaya kosa*, now we are using them about the second sheath, the physiological or organic body, the *pranamaya kosa*. Having strengthened our known selves through asana, we are now adding a second string to our bow through the culture of breath. By so doing, we generate more energy. With more energy we can explore and penetrate further and deeper within.

Whether we are talking about the outermost sheath or this more interior one, we are always bringing the light of awareness. Prana is always involved in carrying that light of awareness, only now we are consciously generating and directing it. In yoga philosophy both energy (prana) and consciousness (*citta*) are considered to evolve directly out of cosmic intelligence (*mahat*). Mahat is the universal intelligence of Nature. The rocks have universal intelligence. Every leaf has it. Every cell of every creature has it. It is all pervasive and infinite. The genius of nature's intelligence is self-expression. That is why nature is infinitely varied, infinitely inventive. Prana is our link to this infinite intelligence. What a shame it is that we have such access and ignore its use and development. We are like someone with a vast fortune locked in a numbered bank account who forgets the number and so must scrape by in poverty. We live within our individual consciousness with its limited intelligence, often feeling lonely and puny, when there is a conduit available directly to cosmic consciousness and intelligence. Through this conduit flows prana, joining each individual among us to the highest original principle of Nature. Pranayama is about restoring this conduit so that the intelligence bearing the energy of the macrocosm can illuminate our microcosm.

Breath and *Pranayama*

I did not start the practice of pranayama until 1944 when I had already been teaching *yogasana* for several years. You can take comfort from the fact that however poor your own pranayama is, it can scarcely be worse than mine was for the first few years. I would wake around four o'clock in the morning and have coffee with my wife. Often I would go right back to sleep. If not, after only three or four minutes, I would start gasping and have to stop. My lung capacity was still impaired from childhood tuberculosis, and in addition I had always overexerted myself in back bends. Through them I had gained suppleness but not the power of resistance. Somehow I persevered. But my chest was taut, and my muscles were sore. Even with my back against a wall, my breathing would be heavy and labored. Gradually I came to realize that whereas back bends strengthen the inner muscles of the spinal column, forward extensions develop its outer muscles. So I did forward bends, timing myself to gain endurance. The pain was intense, like a sledge-hammer hitting my back, and the soreness persisted for hours afterward. I concentrated on twists too, to build up the lateral muscles. It was all very frustrating, and although I avoided the depression that can result from practice, I was terribly restless. You can never do pranayama with an upset mind. Sometimes I used to feel fresh, while at other times I was moody and tense as I never knew how to relax the brain in inhalation or understood the art of the grip needed in the process of exhalation. The grip is the ability to maintain the pranayama posture in a way that allows for inner flexibility and avoids disturbing the posture because of the movement of air. Fortunately, I had the assets of courage and determination in the face of repeated failure.

Initially my guru had told me categorically that I was unfit to do pranayama. In the old days, spiritual knowledge was considered an esoteric subject and jealously guarded by its masters. They were abrupt in their manner and did not think their pupils were deserving enough. One could not talk to them openly and frankly as we do today. Even Ramana Maharishi kept his philosophy for an inner circle of highly qualified scholars. You could say that India at that time was engaged in a struggle for political democracy, but I can assure you that spiritual democracy did not exist. Because I am seen as a stern authoritarian teacher, people do not realize how strongly I have in fact reacted against the harsh and secretive regime in which I was brought up. I am open with everything I have learned, and my strictness has really been a passion for precision so that my students should not suffer from the mistakes and hardship that I had to endure.

Eventually my guru relented to the point where he allowed me to do deep inhalation, retention, and deep exhalation. But he gave no technical instruction. Consequently I was prone to the instability of body and irregular, labored breathing of which Patanjali warns. As I have said, I mercifully escaped the despair or hopelessness that can result, but I was restless and unsettled. Everybody needs a teacher for pranayama. I had no one and fell into the gap between "knowing" and "doing." I *knew* I had to take a deep, slow breath, but it did not happen. I could not *do* it.

It was my asana practice that kept me on track. I continued to adapt and transform my body to be capable of pranayama and so over many long years came to master it. From the point of view of my ability to teach, this process of trial and error has proved a tremendous asset, but it is not a method I would recommend to anyone. My early failures were because of a lack of guidance as well as my own weakness. You, on the other hand, are in a position to build up a good practice in only two or three years, provided you stick with it for as little as ten minutes a day and have a good teacher. As I did, you will learn through action and observation to understand the rising and descending energies of the intelligence and gain the art of surrendering the intelligence and willpower from the seat of the head toward the seat of the heart. By learning how to stretch and how to keep the nervous system elastic and lively through asana, you will be capable of bearing any load, and so stress will not occur at all.

Pranayama is not normal breathing—nor is it just deep breathing. It is the technique of generating cosmic vital energy through the fusion of the antagonistic elements of fire and water. Fire is the quality of mind, and water is the element that corresponds to the physiological body. Water douses fire, and fire evaporates water so they are not easily brought together. Air is the interface whose flow in the lungs provides the dynamic stream that fuses water and fire and produces an energetic current of prana. This spreads through the nervous system and bloodstream and is distributed around the body, rejuvenating every cell. The earth element in the form of body provides the physical location for the production of energy, and the fifth and most subtle element, space or ether, offers the space required for the energy's distribution. The need for a harmonious and symmetrical space explains the importance of the spine and its supporting musculature, for the spine is the central column of the nervous system. By lifting and separating the thirty-three articulations of the vertebral column, and by opening the ribs from the spine like a tiger's claws, we deepen and lengthen the breath.

The analogy of the production of energy through hydroelectric power may prove helpful. Stagnant water can create no energy, which means if you are not breathing, you are dead. If you are breathing normally, there is some flow, and you produce just enough energy for the requirements of the moment. But there is no surplus to be invested in other projects. It is only by the techniques of pranayama, which regulate, channel, and (in retention of breath) dam the flow all the better to harness and extract its inherent power, that we produce sufficient energy to vitalize the whole system. We must live fully before we die. We must generate sufficient energy to realize our full potential. The journey to our infinite core of being is arduous. Only pranic energy can take us there.

Watching the flow of the breath also teaches stability of consciousness, which leads to concentration. There is no finer method. The power of concentration allows you to invest your new energy judiciously. In the yogic scheme of things, the highest application of that concentration and power of vision is in meditation. By learning to appreciate breath, we learn to appreciate life itself. The gift of breath is the gift of life. When we receive a gift, we feel gratitude. Through pranayama we learn gratitude for life and gratitude toward the unknown divine source of life. Let us look now more closely at the movements of breath, their implications and effects.

Yogic breathing techniques are meditative in their origin and in their effect. They basically consist of four parts. They are inhalation (*puraka*), retention of the breath after inhalation (*antara kumbhaka*), exhalation (*recaka*), and retention after exhalation (*bahya kumbhaka*). The in-breath should be long, subtle, deep, rhythmic, and even. The energizing ingredients of the atmosphere percolate into the cells of the lungs and rejuvenate life. By retaining one's in-drawn breath, the energy is fully absorbed and distributed to the entire system through the circulation of blood. The slow discharge of air in exhalation carries out accumulated toxins. By pausing after the out-breath according to one's capacity, all stresses are purged and drained away. The mind remains silent and tranquil. If you over-prolong the pause, you will feel a sudden lurch of panic and suck in more air greedily. This is our instinctive attachment to life reasserting itself. Inhalation is the extension and expansion of the Self (*Purusa*). With the help of the in-breath, the Self embraces its sheaths up to the skin of the body, like a lover embracing his beloved. Retention after inhalation is the union of the lover with his beloved. In exhalation, the Self, via the out-breath, takes the beloved to his home where, in her turn, the beloved embraces her lover, the Self. Retention after exhalation is the beloved uniting with the lover in total surrender to the supreme. Hence, pranayama is more than a physiological breathing exercise. Because breath is life, the art of judicious, thoughtful, ungreedy breathing is a prayer of gratitude we offer to life itself.

It is impossible, when we turn our attention to the inner movement of breath, to use our senses externally at the same time. You cannot also be thinking that you must stop at the supermarket on the way home after work. Pranayama is the beginning of withdrawal from the external engagement of the mind and senses. That is why it brings peacefulness. It is the hinge between extroversion and introversion. When you start asana practice, you gain increased confidence, poise, self-assurance, and the radiance of health. After all, energy is in itself an attractive quality. By all means enjoy these benefits in your contact with the world. But yoga also asks us inwardly to invest some of what we have gained. That is introversion in its positive sense, not a shying away from the world out of feelings of inadequacy, but a desire to explore your inner world. The breath, working in the sheath of the physiological body, serves as a bridge between body and mind.

You cannot look into your mind with your eyes. In asana the eyes should be active to adjust the asana, but in breathing the ears are important in order to listen to the sound of mind's vibration and adjust its harmony. Similarly, the mind too is a vibration in space. The sound of the mind's vibration can be perceived only by the ears. This is the penetration of introspection. It does not bring us closer to the noisy thinking capacity of brain—on the contrary, the organ of brain is pacified. It brings us closer to the intuitive faculty of mind. Nothing pertaining to pranayama can be forced. That is why it teaches humility. So prana itself and its natural companion, the higher intuitive awareness (*prajna*) have to be invited, enticed. When circumstances are favorable, they will come. The metaphor of catching a horse is useful here. You cannot catch a horse in a field by running after it. But if you stand still and hold out an apple, the horse will come to you.

In one sense, the power of will is necessary in pranayama. That is the will of practice, the will to conquer its monotony. Intrinsically it is fascinating, but it offers less variety than asana, and as I have just said, it is an introverted practice. However ardent a practitioner you are, as I was and am myself, do not, however, try to retain the breath by force of will. The moment the brain becomes tense, the inner ears hard, and if the eyes are heavy or irritated throughout, you are forcing beyond your capacity. Be aware of the skin on your trunk that moves toward the inner body. If you know the extension and expansion of the body, you know the extension and expansion of the mind. If the nerves of the body are overloaded, the brain contracts. The sensitivity, the grips, and the stretch of the skin should be like a disciplined child who is both bold and cautious. Let the breath and the intelligence move simultaneously. If the intelligence moves first, you are using force.

Physically, the movements of pranayama involve a vertical ascension, a horizontal expansion, and a circumferential extension of the rib cage, chest wall, and lungs. During inhalation, if the skin over the center of the breastbone can move vertically up and down, and it can expand from side to side circumferentially, it shows that the lungs are being filled to their maximum capacity.

Our normal movement of breath is not rhythmic. Each voluntary inhalation is a stressful action, and each exhalation is nonstressful. Normal involuntary inhalation is not done by the lungs, but by the brain as well as the entire body. One can easily notice that a normal inhalation causes movement in the whole body. The muscles get puffed up, and while exhaling the compression of the muscles can be felt very clearly. In other words, during normal breathing, the entire body inhales, the entire body exhales. In yogic breathing the brain and the extremities of the body remain passive, and only the lungs are activated. The role of the thorax, diaphragm, ribs, intercostal muscles, abdomen, and lungs is therefore different as the breath is received but not sucked in. Because it is the physiological or organic sheath that links and integrates body and mind, it needs to be cultivated with the proper blood and energy supply. In order to affect this, the respiratory system is used totally, but without straining the nervous system.

In normal inhalation, the brain not only draws in the energy, but also the blood. In exhalation it releases it. Such breathing is nothing more than the pumping of blood in and out of the brain. The very word, inspiration, meaning both to breathe in and to grasp a feeling in the form of an idea, expresses the way the brain is charged during inhalation. But this kind of inhalation builds up stress in the brain, as its cells are continuously being inflated and deflated. So instead of becoming energized, both body and brain dissipate the available energy. Pranayama begins with observing the movements of normal breathing and letting them become quiet and soft in such a way that there is no load on the cells of the brain. To accomplish this you have to learn to release the diaphragm. The diaphragm is the medium between the physiological and mental sheaths and in consequence tightens as it records stress and tensions that occur in daily life.

You have to immerse yourself in the in-breaths and out-breaths, and in the naturalness of retention without causing any stress in the brain cells or unnecessary disturbances or jerks to the vital organs and nerves. After all, our nerves are liquid semiconductors, and they do not react well to wild fluctuations of current any more than your computer would. You have to tame your breath to tame your brain. Live from moment to moment absorbed in the unruffled flow of the circular movement of the in- and out-breaths. Its current should be like that of a very full, stately river, whose movements cannot be seen.

If the mind is predominant during inhalation, you are doing egotistical pranayama. If the mind descends, and it is the heart that is predominant, you are doing true, humble pranayama. It is by understanding how to distribute prana that you can bring about the union of the energies of the individual and of the universe. Inhalation engulfs the whole body, expanding from center to periphery. During exhalation, the tide recedes drawing back toward the center. The in-breath is a movement toward the peripheral consciousness; the out-breath moves in to the core of consciousness.

We have seen that as leaves move in the wind, your mind moves with your breath. When breath is regulated and pacified, there is a neutralizing effect on the mind. And when you hold your breath, you hold your soul. By retaining the full in-breath, you hold the divine infinite within yourself. At this moment you have reached the full potential of your individuality, but it is a divine individuality and not the small, selfish creature you normally take yourself for. By exhaling you generously give out your individual self to the universal world. To expire means both to breathe out and to die. What dies is the known I-sense, which clings passionately to its own identity and existence. In retention after exhalation, you experience life after death. The ego's worst fear is confronted and conquered. The veil of illusion that shrouds the "*me*" is lifted.

Inhalation engulfs the whole body with life. Exhalation surrenders that life to the source of life—the Life Giver. The body moves in toward the core of being, like a puppy nestling against its mother, secure and trusting. If retention causes tension or pain in the head, you are holding from the brain, not the lungs. This is egotistical holding. The key to retention is naturalness. Nature is energy. It supplies all our wants. The ego is finite. Nature's energy is infinite. By denying nature, we deny our own energy. Let this ocean of energy bear up the lungs and let it purify the body and refine the consciousness.

It is because of the possibilities that exist in the relationship between prana and citta (consciousness) that the great yogi Svatmarama in the Hatha Yoga Pradipika concludes that breath is the key to ultimate emancipation. In addition, breath builds up the tremendous power needed in the practitioner to face the infinite light when grace dawns. By withdrawing the mind from our senses of perception and organs of action, retention of breath brings consciousness to rest on the lap of the soul. Retention after inhalation is the fulfillment of the individual's potential for divinity. This "cup that is full" rises to merge with universal energy. Exhalation and retention empty the cup of personal potential for divinity in an act of surrender to the cosmic force. This noble act of self-abnegation merges the yogi's identity totally with his divine origin. In this sense, for me, pranayama acts as the *bhakti marga*, which is the great yogic path of devotion, love, and self-surrender. History records that there have been a few individuals who could achieve this leap into an ego-less state by one peerless act of self-renunciation. However, I am sure that in a modern context, when society encourages from infancy the development of the egoic personality, such a transition is impossible without a long, arduous apprenticeship through the living prayer of pranayama.

It is said in the Hatha Yoga Pradipika that the senses are governed by the mind, the mind is governed by the breath, and the breath is governed by the nerves. Our senses inform our mind and give us information about the world around us, but our senses can also control our mind and control us if we are not careful. The yogi learns to use the mind to govern his senses, and he uses his breath to govern the mind. Yet our mind and breath are not always calm and in control. Indeed, they often become agitated as we experience the stresses and strains of life. Indeed, it is this stress that often cuts our breathing short, as our abdomen constricts from anxiousness. This stress stops our breathing and saps our life energy.

Stress

While there has always been stress in the getting and spending of life, today we suffer from so much culturally and personally created stress. The "rat race" has created much unnecessary tension both within and around us. Because of this fast life, we are neglecting the body and the mind. The body and mind are beginning to pull each other in opposite directions, dissipating our energy. We do not know how to recharge our batteries of energy. As a result, we become careless and callous.

Industrial development and urbanization have no doubt triggered a faster life. Science and technology have given us the boons of physical comfort and leisure. But we do not allow our mind to pause and think. We throw ourselves from one endeavor to another, believing that speed and movement is all there is in life. Therefore stress accumulates in the body, producing psychosomatic ailments from stomach ulcers to cardiac arrest. Emotional stresses imprint themselves on the physical, organic, and neurological bodies, just as music is imprinted on a compact disc. Even animals fall sick and die from emotional stress.

We cannot eliminate stress and tension from our lives. That is not the point. Life is of itself stressful. People go to the cinema to relax. But even watching the picture is stressful. In sleep there is also stress: You move from one position to another because of stress. You sit in meditation, and there is stress. If you collapse your spine while meditating, you go to sleep, so you have to keep your spine erect, and that is stressful. Walking, eating, reading—everything is stress. There is nothing in this world free from stress until death. Rather than asking, "Can I be completely free from stress?" we must ask, "What is the degree of stress?" What matters ultimately is how stress affects your nervous system. Positive stress is a measured response to Nature's challenges. It is constructive and does not harm the nerves. But when it is destructive, it is negative stress, which is indeed harmful. In short, our aim is to be able to deal with stress as and when it arises, and not to imprint and accumulate it in the body's various systems, including both conscious and unconscious memory.

Obviously the key to overcoming stress is to calm and strengthen the nervous system. The eyes are so close to the brain that their tension and jitteriness reflects how ragged the nerves have become through overload. Whether your purpose is simply health, or health as a prelude to meditation, these disruptive patterns of energy that we call stress need to be pacified and eliminated from the body. Otherwise progress toward the higher levels of yoga and the more harmonious ways of life will not come.

The main causes of negative stress are anger, fear, speed, greed, unhealthy ambition, and competition, which produce a deleterious effect on the body and mind. When one does good work without selfish motives, though there is the stress of work, it is positive, and it does not cause the far greater stress that comes from grasping and greed. The practice of asana and pranayama not only de-stress you, but energize and invigorate the nerves and the mind in order to handle the stress that comes from the caprices of life.

Consider this analogy. When it rains heavily, the water does not necessarily penetrate the earth. If the surface is dry and hard, the rain water floods the surface and runs off. But if it rains gradually for many days continuously, and the ground is moist, then the water seeps deep into the earth, which is good for cultivation and for life. Similarly in ourselves, we must moisten our muscles and nerves through the expansion and extension of the various asana. In this way, the stress that saturates the brain is diffused throughout the rest of the body, so the brain is rested and released from strain and the body releases its stress and strain through movement. Similarly, while doing the various types of pranayama the whole body is irrigated with energy. The nerves are soothed, the brain is calmed, and the hardness and rigidity of the lungs are loosened. The nerves are made to remain healthy. There is a certain vibration, which you can make rhythmic and subtler in your asana and pranayama practice without force or stress. You are one with yourself and that is in and of itself a meditative state.

This quest for inner peace and contentment through yoga is the solution to the accumulation of stress that we experience in our lives. Two principal practices, yogasana and pranayama, help enormously with stress, but yoga offers a wider solution to stress. The cure to combat the three Ss—stress, strain, and speed—can be found in three Ws—the work of devoted practice, the wisdom that comes of understanding the self and the world, and worship because ultimately surrendering what we cannot control allows the ego to relax and lose the anxiety of its own infinitesimally small self in the infinitude of the divine.

The speed, stress, and strain of modern life send the human system out of gear. The human body is the finest machine created by God. Millions of cells are produced every second and die out just as swiftly. The cells have their own intelligence. They give strength, fitness, and mental calm. The orchestra of bones, muscles, tissues, nerves, blood vessels, limbs, and organs in the circulatory, respiratory, digestive, and glandular systems is tuned to a veritable dance that is sustained by the energy of prana and choreographed by our consciousness. While yoga may begin with the cult of the body, it leads toward the cultivation of our consciousness. As we cultivate our mind, we are able to avoid the stress that would otherwise lodge itself in our body, causing disease and suffering.

As I have said, you must not think that the practice of meditation alone is going to remove stress. Only by learning how to relax the brain can one remove stress. Stress is related to our very nerves and cells. One must learn to calm these cells and cool them down when they overheat with anxious and distracting thoughts. Keeping the brain in a receptive state is the art that yoga teaches. Many people have been taught that meditation is a method of stress relief. In yoga, stress must be dealt with before one can truly begin to meditate. True meditation (*dhyana*) is when the knower, the knowledge, and the known become one. This is only possible when one is in a stress-less state.

Meditation (dhyana) is an essential part of yoga, and potentially there is dhyana in every aspect or petal of yoga. Each one requires a reflective or meditative mood. Meditation is related to the higher mental faculty for which one needs preparation. Learning asanas certainly helps. If I say, "Relax your brain," you cannot do it. If I put you in a certain asana, your brain relaxes, and you become quiet. This is the beauty of yoga. If you do *Halasana* (Plough Pose) your brain becomes completely quiet. If you are dejected mentally, you can do *Setu Bandha Sarvangasana* (a pose in which the body is arched like a bridge) for ten minutes, and your depression disappears, though you do not know how this transformation has occurred. This is how the body is used to cultivate the mind. When the suffering, depressed mind is cured, the light of the soul can itself radiate to the surface of our being.

WHEN YOU ARE EMOTIONALLY DISTURBED, insecurity and anxiety from the conscious mind is converted into the unconscious mind, which is actually hidden in the heart not the brain. Dread of the future, insecurity over whether the necessities and requirements of life will be met and fulfilled or not, and fear of losing what one has are worries that plague people around the world. These worries may come from money, house, job, friends and relatives, and community. Whether from name and fame (work) or near and dear ones (family), we all face the same troubles. Humans innately resist change because we feel safe with what is familiar and fear the insecurity that comes with something new. We tend to live in a familiar fixed routine and try to avoid accepting or even feeling what is beyond the known. But life inevitably oscillates, moves, and changes between the known and the unknown. So often we are not ready to accept the flow of life. We seek freedom but cling to bondage. We do not allow life to "happen" and take on its own shape. Conflicts, opposition, clash of interests and ideas, collision of ego (personal and collective), and limited under-standing are all inevitable parts of life.

The yogic solution to all these vicissitudes is to study how to adapt and build ourselves up. The key is to control the emotional distur-bances and the mental fluctuations. Conscious self-control will save many a situation. When we have done all that can be done, we are ready to face the future fearlessly, and we are able to handle whatever it may bring. We also can control the dualities and conflicts within ourselves. This allows us to reserve all our energies for dealing with life's inevitable challenges, its ups and downs, and its sorrows and joys, with increasing equanimity and less and less emotional upheaval.

The pranamaya kosa, the energetic sheath, is not only where we work with breath but also where we work with our emotions. You have no doubt noticed that your breath is deeply affected by your emotions. Perhaps crying is the most obvious example of how your breathing is altered by your emotions. For any serious work with our breath and with the energy of the body, we must face the six emotional disturbances.

The Six Emotional Disturbances

Through yoga we are able to lessen the six emotional disturbances that cause us so much anguish: lust, pride and obsession, anger, hatred, and greed. They are called negative emotions by Western psychology or deadly sins by Christianity, and indeed these emotional reactions are the enemies of spiritual growth when they are beyond our control. However, each of these emotions exists for a purpose and can be used wisely. For example, the same emotions are transformed and expressed in sentimental terms, gestures, and poses in the composition of Indian Classical dance. Indeed, our feelings have a great deal of energy, which when not directed outward at the world can be cultivated for our Inward Journey.

Religions tell us to get rid of these emotions, but we cannot. They are human emotions that we will feel whether we want to or not. Suppression does not work. George Stevenson invented the steam engine because he noticed that the steam in a boiling kettle lifted the lid. The force was irresistible. Yoga is about channeling and transforming that energy to higher purposes, just as Stevenson used the energy of steam to drive locomotives. There is a saying that war is diplomacy conducted by other means. It would be truer to say that war is greed or pride enacted on the stage of human history. So, since emotions are part of the physiological interface between body and mind, let us look at these six disturbances in greater detail.

Ninety-nine percent of all human communication is emotional, not intellectual. Emotions, far more than thoughts, guide most behavior in the world. Emotions relate not only to what we feel, but to the value we place on things. Human life is concerned very much with exchanges, and when we disagree about the value of what we are exchanging, misunderstanding and disharmony can ensue. To understand the emotions, we have to recognize the role the ego plays in them, which I shall explain later. In these emotional disturbances most people become stuck and find themselves bouncing from one to the other like billiard balls. Yoga helps in allowing us to get off this emotional pool table. It teaches us how to control our emotions so they do not control us. In this way, we can sublimate them and become masters of our circumstances and not slaves to them.

In our spiritual quest, it is required of us that we develop our body in such a way that it is no longer a hindrance, a drag, but becomes our friend and accomplice. Similarly, our emotions and intellect must be developed for divine purposes. Since we all suffer from them, yoga tends to see them as sicknesses of mind, inherent problems that devolve from the human condition itself. After all, you do not blame someone who lives in a tropical swamp when he catches malaria. You simply look for ways to cure him. The man is not evil, the mosquito is only doing what mosquitoes do, and the swamp is probably rich in food and life or else no one would live there. So it is not a question of looking for blame, but looking for a solution.

Suppose you own a car that has difficulty starting on cold mornings. You cannot afford a better car, but you do know that if you take the trouble to spread a tarpaulin on the hood on cold nights, the car will function perfectly in the morning. In other words, your car has a weakness, a defect, but with a little forethought and trouble, it will not cause a problem. That is the attitude we should have toward the six emotional disturbances. As the modern saying goes, we should live in the solution, not in the problem.

Most Westerners try to solve their emotional problems through intellectual understanding. Emotional issues can, however, be resolved only through emotional understanding. Emotions lie in a physical sense in the organs of the physiological body—at the level of the pranamaya kosa. Think of the irritable, liverish army colonel who abuses his liver with too much chili and brandy. So too, our positive, beneficial emotions have their seat in healthy organs. It is the health of the physiological body that creates the primary link between Health and Salvation. Look at children; they are innocent because they are organically healthy. The two go together. World-weary organs indulge in world-weary vice.

I have said that emotions have their root in the organic body, but they do not always stay there. They invade and occupy memory. A dog can feel angry, but only we humans can say, "I am so angry with my boss," and record it in memory. When we say we feel angry, it is a mental perception of our state, and having registered that perception, we record it in memory where it becomes part of the stock and furniture of mind. The dog might subsequently come across the sensory stimulus that brings back the anger, or fear, or whatever the emotion is, but that is a cellular memory, a conditioned reflex, absent when the trigger that fires it is not activated. The point about us is that we carry around within the recollection of mind our rancor, resentments, hates, greed, and lust, even when the motivating stimulus is absent. So when our boss is on holiday, we carry on hating him. This does not harm him, but it certainly pollutes and poisons us. It is both a blockage and a dissipation of our vital energies. Who is rich enough to afford such waste? Who is pure enough to endure such systemic toxin?

To feel is a verb; it is something that happens. We all feel. Emotion is a noun, a thing. To feel is beautiful, belonging to both the animal and human condition. When we allow feelings to harden and coalesce into emotions, which we transport like overburdened slaves, we deny ourselves life's freshness, its ever-present potential for renewal and transformation. We waste so much energy through allowing our emotions to govern us. Feelings and emotions involve our organs, breath, and mind. Those feelings that we experience before they pop up in our heads are called "gut" feelings and are respected for their instinctual source. In a healthy organism, feelings should pass like clouds over the sun. When feelings get anchored by thought into our memory, they become emotions, which are no longer related to the moment but to the past. They accrue a greater density and darkness, like storm clouds that block out the sun itself. These stagnant emotions poison us and prevent us from seeing what truly is.

Look at your dog. When you leave him, he is sad; his heart is on the ground. When you come home, is there resentment? No, he is overjoyed to see you. Are you closer to reality or is your dog?

Normally, we find life full of pressure, pain, tension, stress, and strain. By understanding these six emotional disturbances that plague humanity, we will be able to have a chance at transforming them and transforming ourselves.

Lust

Nothing scatters the mind more than lust. Yet lust is the impetus for procreation. It is the glue that holds family life together. Sexual dissatisfaction is where problems in marriage begin. Patience and tolerance are necessary. There is a natural progression in marriage whereby the importance of passion becomes less important—not unimportant, but less important—and its place is filled evermore by love and friendliness. The gateway to divine love, I believe, as I have experienced it, is through personal love—the love of one other incarnate soul. Just as you cannot find illumination by jumping from one guru to another, according to your whims, you will not easily find the greater love of God if you keep on finding imperfections in particular creations. By and large, and I acknowledge cultural differences, there is merit in sticking with what you have started. I have admitted that pranayama can be boring. To a scattered mind, so can sexual fidelity. But to love One is to access All. Trust and faith bind us not only to each other but to the Universal. When the breath is gently exhaled towards the heart, the heart is purified of desires and the emotions that disturb it. The Love that transcends the particularity of individual attraction and perceives the soul within the other is the great pathway to God.

Of course, it is easy to say this aged eighty-six. When I was a young man, I had to fight to keep my integrity. Virtue is an ideal. Integrity is a reality. I did not want to divide myself. The *di* root in Sanskrit is the same as division and devil in English. It implies fragmentation and loss of self. I knew that if I had ceded to the temptation of a prostitute as a young man, I would have had to marry her or lose my integrity. In an angry moment, I even wrote that to my guru, when I was falsely accused of immorality. The great nineteenth-century saint, Ramakrishna, fell into a state of *samadhi* when he was introduced to prostitutes, as all he could perceive was the Goddess within them.

Later on, when I was married and teaching abroad, I was exposed to temptation. It is normal for women students to set their teacher on a pedestal in any subject, but by that time I was a bit more worldly-wise and developed a forbidding manner to keep them at arm's length. My flashing eyebrows and fierce glare came to my rescue.

Sensual desire when joined with love is an important part of a marriage. I had a passionate marriage, and if my wife, Ramamani, was alive today the intensity of our feelings would be undimmed. Often one partner in a marriage will pursue yoga or another spiritual path, and they will leave the other partner behind. They must not. They must do whatever they have to in order to bring the other partner along or to always return to the other partner. This is the only way to keep the marriage strong.

Sexuality is natural and sacred, as is all the natural world. It is the way we use, channel, and direct it that makes the difference between the sacred and the profane, between the augmentation of devotion and what Shakespeare described in his sonnet, "The expense of spirit in a waste of shame is lust in action."

Yoga does not use the word power very often. Yet it is implicit in all mention of ego. The ego seeks power because it seeks self-perpetuation; it seeks at all costs to avoid its own inevitable demise. To achieve that impossible end, it devises a thousand ruses. Sexuality is essentially the beauty of birds nesting in spring. Is this nature's joy or is it sin? But what has ego done to procreation, to the harmonious union of complementary opposites? It has twisted it into an act of egoic self-affirmation. Lust is self-validation through consumption. Control through the exercise of power. When the emergence of human ego came into the world, it altered the act of procreation. It converted it to an existential proof of being through an act of consumption, not consummation.

Pride and Obsession

The problem with all six emotional disturbances is when ego becomes involved with them. Without ego, you can hate injustice, as Gandhi did in South Africa. Without ego, you can take pride in accomplishment. Yehudi Menuhin was humble before his art, as I am before mine, but that does not deprive us of the right to pride of achievement. Simply we do not attach it to ego; it is a gift that we have been given the grace to share. Obsession can be translated as infatuation or addiction—all states in which the ego is in bondage. Fanaticism is another word for obsession. Yehudi Menuhin and I both practiced our art fanatically.

But were we fanatics? Not to other people. Our ego had no attachment to forcing and controlling others. A passion for excellence is one thing; to force one's beliefs and practices down other people's throats is another. That is ego; that is pride.

The yoga path is not easy and requires almost a commitment that to many may seem extreme or even fanatical. I am fanatical with myself when I practice yoga. It is true. You should be fanatical with yourself but not with others. My guru was fanatical with everyone including me. He applied his standards to everyone. I try to know my students' abilities and to help them to reach their highest potential, not mine. I shall deal with ego and pride more fully in chapter 5 as they form part of the five afflictions that are central to any understanding of yoga. Obsession in the sense of addictive patterns of behavior is dealt with fully in chapter 4.

Anger

We have all seen when anger is out of control or destructive. Husband and wife shout at each other in the bedroom; drivers yell at each other in the street. Anger is out of control when it flares up in us like a fire that we have no control over and that smolders long after the fire is out. We shout and call people names and say things we might not even mean because we are in a rage. We continue to be resentful and to ruminate on the offense we have received long after. This is anger that comes from our ego. Another car cuts us off in the street, and we feel offended. "He cut *me* off!" we tell ourselves. He did this to *me*. He has offended *me*. He has affronted my ego.

As we practice yoga and begin to meditate, we develop equanimity. We let go of this ego. We realize that most of life is not personal. The driver was not trying to cut us off because he did not have respect for us. We realize that it had nothing to do with us. As our minds grow quieter, our first thought is not, "That idiot!" Instead we think to ourselves, perhaps he was rushing to the hospital to see his dying parent. In the West, people take everything very personally and so there is even now something called Road Rage where drivers will attack and even shoot each other. In Pune and most of India, we still do not have traffic lights, and our streets are a throng of drivers, pedestrians, and sometimes animals all trying to cross each other and only narrowly avoiding each other. Drivers honk their horns constantly at each other to alert each other that they are there and to vie for position, but we take it far less personally. We know that it is the roads and millions of people trying to live their lives and get to where they are going. This does not mean that we do not have traffic disputes or go to court when we crash. Every Indian is not a yogi, but our culture reminds us that sometimes life is impersonal. We all are subject to impersonal forces—like traffic.

Often people say that I have a temper because I will shout at people in class when I see that they are putting themselves at risk or conversely not doing their best. For this reason people have said that I am a severe teacher. I am strict, but I am not harsh. I use my anger to free a student from his pattern. One student kept talking about his fear in *Sirsasana*, and I finally shouted, "Forget about fear. You may only fall on the floor, not beyond. In the future there is fear. In the present there is no fear." He was startled, but he got the point. A commander in the army who is heading into battle can not always speak softly to his soldiers. Sometimes he must shout at them to motivate them quickly, and sometimes he must speak gently to give them courage. The battle of yoga is with the body and with the ego. You must conquer your ego, or small self, so that you can let your soul, your big Self, be victorious.

A young boy was brought to me by his parents. For weeks he had been in a daze, like a trance. I sent the parents away and asked him what was wrong. He told me that the divine *Kundalini* energy had been awakened in him. Kundalini energy is very sacred and very rare.

It is as if he had said he had been enlightened. I slapped him across the face. I knew he was deluded and simply tricking his parents for whatever reason he had. At first he was startled, but he paid attention, and then I showed him how to do a number of asanas that helped to ground him and bring him to himself. I am not suggesting that teachers should hit their students or that parents should hit their children. Too often this is done because the teacher or parent is out of control, and this is destructive anger. I am saying that there is a place for righteous anger—not self-righteous anger—that we use skillfully in a way that helps rather than hurts others. I was not angry with the boy. I was angry with his delusion. The slap was to awaken him from his dangerous fantasy. Perhaps the simplest and most common example is when a mother grabs her small child as he is stepping into the street. The mother's anger is constructive, and she may scold the child to make sure the child learns how to stay safe. If the mother ruminates on her anger and continues to shout at the child all day, it is not constructive, for the child will think that the mother is angry with *him* and not simply with what he has done.

Hatred

Hatred and its relatives, malice and envy, are the last of the emotional disturbances mentioned by Patanjali. The destructive nature of hatred is everywhere evidenced in intolerance, violence, and war. But it also exists in our own lives when we wish others ill or envy what they have. If they are less, we feel like we are more. There is a story about a farmer who encounters a great magician who tells him he can have anything he wants. The farmer's reply is that he wants his neighbor's cow to die. The offices of psychiatrists in the West are filled with adults whose parents loved one child in the family more than the other, causing hatred and sibling rivalry in the family. As we see in this example, even something like a parents love can be destructive. We must use our intelligence with all of our emotions, not just the negative ones.

And yet even with hatred there is a positive. When I invited sex and drug addicts to live in my house to cure them of their problem, I hated their addiction. I hated what it did to them and how it ruined their lives. A wise teacher can use their hatred of their students' faults to correct them and help them. Insecure or depressed students may not at first see this advice as constructive, thinking to themselves, "My teacher hates me." But eventually they will see that the teacher, if the teacher has used his intelligence, was trying to help them.

Greed

I have always been a man of appetite and enthusiasm. In my youth I was often hungry, but on one glorious occasion I entered and won a *jalebi* eating competition. Jalebis are a rich, heavily sugared batter, deep fried in *ghee* (clarified butter). I ate seventy-six jalebis. While I can still stand on my head for twenty minutes, I don't think I could still eat seventy-six jalebis. Appetite for life is wonderful—for scents, for sights, for taste, and for color and human experience. You just have to learn to control it. Quality is more important than quantity. Take in the essence of life as you would smell the fragrance of a flower, delicately and deeply, with sensitivity and appreciation.

If appetite is a gift, and greed a sin, then waste is a crime. We waste our food, our energy, our time, our lives. We seek power from the accumulation of surplus; we are greedy for more than our fair share. In a finite world, we search for infinite satiation. Will more money than we can spend in a lifetime prolong that life? Can we eat a larder full of food when we are dead? The villain is the ego. He has read the law of intensification, which says that more is better, and we shall see more of his tricks in the next chapter. Our planet groans under the burden of this greed.

The ways in which our greed are destructive in our world are easy to see. The ways in which our greed is destructive in our lives is more difficult. When we are greedy, we are never satisfied, and we are never content. We are always afraid that there will not be enough, and we become miserly. Instead of seeing our riches and giving generously to others, we become nothing more than rich beggars, always asking for more. In yoga we consciously minimize our needs. We do this not to show how holy we are because we can live on a few grains of rice. We minimize our needs so that we can minimize our attachments and to maximize our contentment. In so doing we are able to lessen our greediness. For one man a meal is slight; for another it is a feast. Life is the same way. The fewer our demands on life, the greater is our ability to see its bounty.

I was once asked to teach yoga to a very wise man while I was in Europe. He was revered around the world for his wisdom and his holiness. However, this man had a weakness for cars. Despite the fact that he was living off of the generosity of others, he was willing to accept a gift from one of his devotees of a Rolls Royce race car that was a two-seater. Someone had driven me in this car once, and I knew it was a nice one, but it was a very expensive one too. His devotee told me that he had sold his home in order to buy this car. Because I do not hide my feelings, I told this man that I thought he was wrong to accept it. I told him that I was happy with my cotton shirts, but he needed his silk ones. This does not make me holier than him. It just makes my needs less and my ability to be content greater. I watched this revered teacher each day polishing his car himself for two hours because he did not want anyone else to touch it. This man's love of cars and need for this car was a trap that made him greedy.

Greed, however, is not just for possessions. We can be greedy for affection or attention just as easily. Some time after the man received this two-seater, one of his other devotees bought him a new Mercedes race car that was a four-seater. This student wanted desperately to be closer to his teacher and thought that if there were more seats in his car than he could drive around with him as well. I tell my students that anyone who thinks that they are closer to me than anyone else has understood nothing about yoga. Our greed comes from our fear that we will not have enough—whether it is money or love that we grasp. Yoga teaches us to let go of these fears and so to realize the abundance around us and within us.

REMEMBER THAT YOGA IS NOT ASKING us to refrain from enjoyment. Draw in the exquisite fragrance of the flower. Yoga is against bondage. Bondage is being tied to patterns of behavior from which we cannot withdraw. Repetition leads to boredom, and eventually boredom is a form of torture. So yoga says keep the freshness, keep the pristine, keep the virginity of sensitivity. By all means, as I have suggested, keep an eye on our capricious ego, but there are techniques beyond that. The aim of retention (*kumbhaka*) is to restrain the breath. While breath is being held, speech, perception and hearing are controlled. The citta (consciousness) in this state is free from passion and hatred, greed and lust, pride and envy. Prana and citta become one in retention. Citta wavers with the breath, while retention frees it from desire. Patanjali also describes other means to address the Emotional Disturbances and other obstacles that we find on our Inward Journey, which we will now explore.

To begin with, there is an important point to be made about these inner conflicts, or Emotional Disturbances. They cannot be conquered without discretion (*vivecana*). But in order to be victorious over the six causes of delusion or emotional disturbances, one has to use the six spokes of the wheel of peace. These are: discrimination and reasoning, practice and detachment, and faith and courage. To distinguish pleasant transient sensations from permanent spiritual delights, discrimination and reasoning (*viveka* and *vicara*) are required. They have to be developed through practice (*abhyasa*) and detachment (*vairagya*). Practice involves *tapas* (the purifying fire of action). Tapas is nothing but disciplining the mind through the eight limbs of yoga. This practice is not complete without faith (*sraddha*) and courage (*virya*). These should be combined with the study of sacred texts and of one's own behavior (*svadhyaya*), determination (*drdhata*), and meditation (dhyana). In order to gain clarity and calmness of mind, it is particularly pranayama that has the power to calm the ruffled and vagrant mind.

I have said that the cure for our inherent flaws lies in sustained practice of the eight petals of yoga. Knowledge of yoga is no substitute for practice. Since the difficulties lie within ourselves, so do the solutions. Nevertheless, Patanjali in his compassion and wisdom offered us a series of specific aids and remedies, which in a very subtle and penetrating way act to reform the afflicted consciousness itself. They are of a refined common sense. These Healthy and Healing Qualities (*vrttis*) are like a balm we can rub on our skin that gradually penetrates the skin, muscles, and fiber and relieves the deep pain within.

The Healthy *Vrttis*

The first specific advice that Patanjali gives us about these disturbances I will translate very loosely. "If you are happy, pleasant, and unselfish in your behavior toward others, obstacles will shrink. If you are miserly with your emotions and judgmental in your mind, obstacles will grow." More precisely, what Patanjali said is this. In order to achieve a serene consciousness, we have to be willing to change our behavior and approach toward the external world. This is for our own good. Certain treatments, known as the Healthy and Healing Qualities of Consciousness, cultivate the mind and smooth the yogic path. They are:

1. *Maitri*—Cultivation of friendliness toward those who are happy.

2. *Karuna*—Cultivation of compassion toward those who are in sorrow.

3. *Mudita*—Cultivation of joy toward those who are virtuous.

4. *Upeksa*—Cultivation of indifference or neutrality toward those who are full of vices.

These four seem so simple as to be banal. In reality they are subtle and deep. Remember that I opened the discussion of emotional disturbances by treating them as naturally occurring flaws by which we dissipate our energies. In other words, energy must be enticed within, increased through techniques of generation, contained, distributed, and invested within. But in reality we leak energy like a sieve. Whenever you are jealous of someone else's happiness and fortune, you leak energy. "It should have been me," you say. "Why did he win the lottery, not me?" Jealousy, envy, and resentment impoverish the person who feels them, not just morally but energetically. They literally shrink you. To take joy in the well-being of others is to share in the riches of the world. When we dip our cup into the infinite, we are enriched, but the infinite is not diminished. When you stare at the sunset, you are filled with its beauty, but the sunset remains as beautiful as ever. When you resent the happiness of others, you lose even the little that you have.

Worse than that, when you are puritanical toward the defects you perceive in others, when you are condemnatory and disdainful toward the victims of vice and use their misfortune to feel superior, you are playing a dangerous game. "There but for the grace of God, go I" should be your attitude. Otherwise you are setting yourself up for a fall. Besides which, it is exhausting to spend one's time disapproving of others. It causes your ego to form a hard shell of false pride and certainly has no reforming effect on the victim of your disapprobation. Compassion for the suffering of others is more than just sympathy. The superficial sympathy we express for the woes of others, when we watch the nightly television news, for example, is often no more than a wish to feel good about ourselves, a sop to our own conscience. "I am a person of sensibility and feeling," we say. Without action, this is mere self-indulgence.

It is a modern illusion to imagine that positive emotions, sympathy, pity, kindness, and a general but diffused goodwill are the equivalent of virtues. These "soft" emotions can serve as a form of narcissistic self-indulgence. Often they are impotent. They make us feel good about ourselves, like when we give a coin to a beggar. They create the illusion of health and well-being. But sensitivity should be used as a diagnostic tool, not as a mirror to our own vanity. Real compassion is potent as it implies the question, "What can I do to help?" The compassion Mother Teresa of Calcutta felt for the dying and dispossessed was always a spur to action, to care, to intelligent intervention.

Positive emotions are not the same as virtue. Virtue is valor, moral courage, persistence in adversity, and protection of the weak against the tyranny of the strong—not hand-wringing sympathy. Compassion is the recognition of sameness, of kinship with others. It is potent and practical. Alcoholics, drug addicts, and sex addicts were welcome to use my house as a safe haven until their cravings subsided to a manageable level. For fifty odd years, I have given several medical classes a week for the most intractable cases. I am glad for the benefit that this has given my patients. I am equally glad for the benefit it has brought me—the opportunity to meet and greet the godhead within each man, woman, and child and with openness, energy, and ingenuity to try to palliate their sorrows. Similarly the virtue of others is not a reproach to our own inadequacy, but an uplifting example to us. Not only the great, like Gandhiji, fulfill this role. If you watch a sportsman who has won a cup speak of his victory with modesty and gratitude and with generosity toward his adversaries, is not his virtuous behavior a feast for you also? These healing qualities are jewels that bring grace to our consciousness and life.

Pranayama—our breath—can also help. We can bring calmness

and quietness to our minds and our emotions with the retention of breath after exhalation. I have said that exhalation empties the brain and pacifies the ego, bringing it to quiescent humility. When you empty the brain, you also empty the toxins of memory. With an exhalation and retention, you let go of resentment, anger, envy, and rancor. Exhalation is a sacred act of surrender, of self-abandonment. At the same time we abandon all those stored up impurities that cling to the self— our resentments, angers, regrets, desires, envies, frustrations, and feelings of superiority and inadequacy and also the negativity that causes the obstacles to adhere to consciousness. When ego falls away, they fall away with it. Of course they return, but the remembered experience of peace acts as proof that these obstacles are not insurmountable; they can be detached and disposed of. Ultimately they are not permanent and integral to consciousness but ailments that can be cured. We carry so many toxins in memory, feelings that we have stored away and allowed to stagnate and fester. We get so used to carrying this sack of rubbish around that we even conclude it is just part and parcel of our character.

There is something called "echo" exhalation that impresses this point even further. Exhale slowly and fully. Pause. Then exhale again. There is always a slight residue left in the lungs. In that residue is to be found the sludge of toxic memory and ego. In that brief further exhalation, let them go—and experience an even deeper state of relief from burden, of peace and emptiness. In inhalation we experience the full "I," human potential fulfilled and raised like a brimming cup in offering or oblation to the Cosmic Divine. In exhalation we experience the empty "I," the divine void, a nothingness that is complete and perfect, a death that is not the end of life. Try it. Exhale slowly and fully. Pause. Then exhale again.

A practical illustration of how exhalation helps us to calm disturbance and overcome sorrow is that when someone has received a shock or bad news, we often say to them, "Take a deep breath." The point of this is that a deep in-breath produces a deep, full exhalation, and it is this that produces the calming and quietening effect you want on the disturbed person.

Another cure that Patanjali suggests is to contemplate an object that helps to maintain steadiness of mind and calm the consciousness. From the yogic point of view, this technique should be considered as a sort of healing meditation. I will give non-yogic examples of this so that you can see its foundation in good sense. When you are ill in bed and feeling miserable, if you read a good, serious, interesting, absorbing book, your concentration brings about a steadiness of mind that relieves you from the distress of illness and helps the healing process. All illness fragments and so whatever integrates also heals. It is axiomatic in yoga that illness has its origin in the consciousness. Self-cultivation really begins only with total self-absorption, so anything that facilitates concentration, reflection, and inward absorption is going to begin to heal the problems of the fissured, imbalanced self.

A further remedy is to contemplate a sorrowless inner light. Yet this form of meditation can occur almost spontaneously in the terminally sick. This vision of where they are going can bring relief and reconciliation in acute suffering.

Yet another remedy is contemplating divine or enlightened sages. In western culture that may seem an odd remedy for illness or anguish, but until modern times often the only recourse of the sick was to turn in prayer and devotion to the saints like Saint Bernadette of Lourdes. Though cultural forms differ, there is a universal, perennial wisdom operating here. When we contemplate those who have the qualities that we aspire to, we move closer to those qualities.

The final healing suggestion is to recollect in wakefulness a calm, dreamless, or dream-filled sleep. The point about all of these is that they are forms of auto-suggestion, taking an auspicious object of contemplation that is calmer, more tranquil, and more enduring and elevated than we are, and by that contemplation aligning our own mind with that more peaceful and collected state.

As we begin to withdraw our ego and the attachment to our feelings that disturb us, as we use the Healing Qualities to calm our hearts and minds, we also begin to withdraw from the vicissitudes of life. This withdrawal is called *Pratyahara*. It is an important part of experiencing inner peace.

Pratyahara

Earlier we examined pranayama, the fourth petal of the flower of yoga. We have seen that it creates energy and purifies the body and its organs and functions. It even calms the six emotional disturbances. I also mentioned that when we turn our attention fully to the inner movement of breath, our senses lose their acuity in relation to the external world. This is in the same way that when we are concentrating on writing an essay for school or university, we cease even to be aware of the road work going on in the street. Though asana practice takes one's mind to peep inside the body, it is in pranayama that one begins to learn to withdraw the senses and mind from their external engagement. By this the awareness and energy are invested *within*. This is the opposite of what happens when you are having a hectic day at the office.

The fifth petal of yoga (pratyahara) is a continuation and intensification of this process, leading to mastery of mind and senses. I said that for a beginner, exertion through sweat is greater than the penetration to one's core, and that in pranayama penetration gathers momentum. I called it a hinge. In the same way, pratyahara is considered to be a hinge or pivotal movement on yoga's path, when the energies created by practice (abhyasa) need to be matched and balanced by the prudence of detachment (vairagya). Practice generates a centrifugal force, a spinning and expanding energy. Trouble comes when this compelling energy spins out of control. Military training works in the same way, which is why soldiers on leave and sailors on shore so often get into trouble. Military discipline and honor are their safeguards. Detachment is the disciplinary safeguard of the yoga practitioner. It is a centripetal force that reinvests, with unswerving purpose, the strengths and abilities we have gained toward the search for the core of being. This voluntary self-discipline is the role of pratyahara. Without it, the yoga practitioner, whose body and spirit are strengthened, will waste his or her efforts and become enamored with the greater attention or attraction they receive from the world.

In Sanskrit, pratyahara literally means "to draw toward the opposite." The normal movement of the senses is to flow outward where they encounter the objects of the world and name and interpret them with the aid of thought. These thoughts will probably be of acquisition (I want), rejection (I don't want), or resignation (there's nothing I can do about it). Rain, for example, will on different occasions elicit all three responses. Pratyahara, then, implies going against the grain, a difficult retraction, which is why it is often compared to a tortoise drawing his head, tail, and four limbs back inside his shell. The yogi simply observes the fact. "It is raining," he may think or say, without desire or judgment.

You can see how difficult this is by the simple exercise of going for a walk and at the same time trying not to comment on, judge, or even name, what you see, hear, or smell. If you see a motor car, you might find the words "new," "beautiful," "expensive," or "ostentatious" jumping unbidden into your mind. Even on a country walk, though you might be able to stop yourself from saying "beautiful" or "lovely" as a commentary, it will be almost impossible not to let yourself name the objects—teak tree, cherry tree, violet, hibiscus, thorn bush, etc. This almost unstoppable taxonomical impulse demonstrates how we always go out to meet things. We are not naturally receptive and polite. We do not let the sunset come to us and greet it with soft, receptive eyes. Our eyes are hard and shiny and acquisitive as if life were a nonstop shopping spree. Paradoxically our desire to control by description, interpretation, and consumption robs us of much of the scent, taste, and beauty of life. The ability to withdraw our senses and so control the noisy mind may sound like a kill-joy, but in reality it restores the pristine flavors, textures, and discoveries that we associate with the innocence and freshness of childhood. This is truly an example of "less is more," as overindulgence can only dull and exhaust the senses.

The yogic purpose of pratyahara is to make the mind shut up so we can concentrate. As long as the senses pester us for their gratification, we will never get a moment to ourself, or in the sense of our inner quest, Ourself. It is a long and patience-demanding apprenticeship in detachment. A witty man once joked that the only way to get rid of temptation was to give in to it. We all theoretically know the falsity of that, but simply to avoid giving in to desires does not of itself make desire go away. Most of us pretend to ourselves that when we have reasonable self control, we have conquered desire. This is wishful thinking. The absence of vice is a step toward virtue, not virtue itself. Yoga situates the organ of virtue (*dharmendriya*) or conscience, in the heart, and it must be pure. Age, for example, may diminish our capacity for vicious action, but not for vicious thought or intention. Wars may be fought by young men, but they are started by old ones.

Nor does retiring to a cave in the Himalayas make desires disappear. Far from it. It merely makes their gratification extremely problematic. Solitariness and simplicity of life do make us aware of desire as a mental phenomenon in itself, regardless of whether objects of sensory gratification are visible or available. The early Christian saint St. Anthony underwent his great temptations in the Egyptian desert. They tormented him. By this austerity he brought himself face to face with the root of desire itself. This sort of extreme practice has always been common in India too. Patanjali recognized that the higher you rise, the harder you fall. Temptations of a quality one might even describe as celestial should come as no surprise to the higher practitioner, nor should he greet them with attachment. The Sirens do not easily abandon their song. The nearer the victory, the more bitter the battle. Senses that have trained on greed are bound to suffer eventually from indigestion. So we have to make them go on a fast to rejuvenate them. In this way we tame the senses and the mind, actually enhancing their intrinsic qualities. Because it is not extreme there is no backlash. It is the gradual involution of the sense and stilling of the mind with the aid of breath to make the practitioner fit for concentration and meditation. Involution means "turning in." It is not rupture. A student once recited the phrase from a poem "As though a rose should be shut and be a bud again." This is an apt description of pratyahara.

The role of breath is capital for this reason. Consciousness (citta) and vital energy (prana) are in constant association. Where consciousness is focused, there must be the energy of prana too, and where you direct the energy of prana, consciousness follows. Consciousness is propelled by two powerful forces, energy (prana) and desires (*vasana*). It moves in the direction of whichever force is most powerful. If breath (prana) prevails, then desires are controlled, the senses are held in check, and the mind is pacified. If the force of desire gets the upper hand, the breathing becomes uneven, and the mind becomes agitated. These are things you can actually observe, just as you observe right measure and balance in asana, and this is why and where the practice of yoga brings self-knowledge (svadhyaya). You will not reach Knowledge of the Divine Self without passing through self-knowledge. Your practice is your laboratory, and your methods must become ever more penetrating and sophisticated. Whether you are in asana or doing pranayama, the awareness of the body extends outward, but the senses of perception, mind, and intelligence should be drawn inward.

This is pratyahara where sustained practice (tapas) and self-knowledge (svadhyaya) blend together. Traditionally self-knowledge starts with reading scriptures, knowing their meaning and seeing their truths reflected in one's own life. This also includes the teachings of a wise master or guru. It continues and deepens through the self-culture of asana and pranayama practice where one has to be able sensitively to verify differences in actions and make adjustments. Later on one learns to watch the mind itself and its movements and ultimately to keep it stable and quiet. But even here there is danger, for when mind and senses are controlled, the ego itself, like a cobra, raises its hood and hisses. The ego can become inflated, even intoxicated with its own prowess in mind control. Only the next petal of yoga, concentration (*dharana*), which I will look at in chapter 5, will release the knowledge that can truly be called wisdom.

I said earlier that much of human life depends upon exchange; we exchange labor, money, goods, emotions, and affections. This system of exchange also operates within us. In modern terms you might call this form of internal cooperation a feedback system, or interpenetration of one level by another, or of one bodily system by another in mutual support and interdependence. The whole body, what we called in chapter 3 the physical sheath (annamaya kosa), is in reality also penetrated by energy and mind, which are the second and third sheaths. All three levels are dependant on the food we eat, the water we drink, and the air we breathe. Look at the liver for instance. It is a vital organ, so we nourish it with food, but we also enrich it with prana provided we manipulate it properly through extension, contraction, and inversion. This rejuvenating action cannot happen unless the mind also goes there. When we act by applying the mind, the avenue of blood circulation changes too. Through prana, even the chemical properties of the blood can change. Do not think, therefore, that asana pertains only to the physical sheath. There is a total involvement between the three sheaths of body (annamaya kosa), energy (pranamaya kosa), and mind (*manomaya kosa*).

The techniques of yoga give you the opportunity to capture energy from the outside as well as from the inside and to use that energy for your personal evolution. The practice of asana clears the inner channels for prana to move freely and uninterruptedly. If the nerves are corroded and blocked with stress, how can prana circulate? Asana and pranayama practice removes the partition that segregates body and mind. Together they dispel darkness and ignorance. In a sense, it is asana practice that opens the gateway to perfection. It breaks the rigidity and hardness of the inner body. This allows the unrhythmic breath to become rhythmic, deep, slow, and soothing. Then pranayama, in its turn, clears and soothes the feverish brain, making way for reason and clarity of thought and lifting the mind toward meditation.

The sustained practice of pranayama liberates one from fear, including even the fear of death. If there is anxiety in the body, the brain contracts. When the brain relaxes and empties itself, it lets go of its fears and desires. It dwells neither on the past, nor the future, but inhabits the present. Freedom is about dropping the shackles of fear and desire. When freedom comes, there is no anxiety, no nervousness. That means there is no load on the nerves or, through them, on the unconscious mind. By removing tension from the inner layers of the nervous system, you convert them into a state of freedom. When we looked at pratyahara, we saw that freedom offers us choice—either to go on as before, driven by external forces and gratifications, or to turn inward and use our gentle powers to seek out the Self.

When I was a young man in Pune, the Christian community used to sing a hymn. It says, "As pants the hart for cooling streams, when heated in the chase, so pants my soul, oh Lord, for Thee, and Thy refreshing grace." This describes the motivation and inspiration for pratyahara.

Many ask me whether pranayama, controlling the breath, postpones old age. Why worry about it? Death is certain. Let it come when it comes. Just keep working. The Soul has no age. It doesn't die. Only the body decays. And yet, we must never forget the body, since it is the garden we must cherish and cultivate. As we shall see in the next chapter on mind, even something as subtle as mind depends on health and energy, and they start in the garden of the body.

Prana is the great life force of the universe. There is a witness inside us all that we call the Seer or the Soul. To remain in the body, even this seer depends on breath. They arrive together at birth, and they leave together, departing at death. The Upanishads say that these are the only indispensables of life. This is true, for I am reminded of an old man who for thirty years or more sat in the main street of Pune and cleaned shoes. He was terribly crippled, with withered sticks for legs folded on a little wooden trolley. In his youth he was destitute and in despair. Survival seemed impossible. Then one day he began to clean shoes. He had a good chest and gradually his arms strengthened. He was not only the best shoe cleaner in the town, but he was respected and held in friendship by all who passed. The newspapers wrote an article about him, and in old age he even found a suitable wife as a companion. All he had was a fine chest, prana, sparkling wise eyes reflecting the seer within, and his shoe cleaning equipment. The Upanishad was right. With just breath and soul and courage, the man achieved a life to be admired.

So often what prevents us from living an admirable life is the chattering of our minds, which pester us with long outdated doubts and despair. Our minds are truly one of the greatest creations in God's world, but they are so easily disoriented and set spinning. In the next chapter, we explore the beginnings of how our minds work and how learning to cultivate our consciousness through understanding and relearning serves as the key for our emancipation.

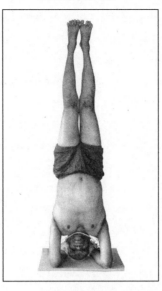

Chapter 4

CLARITY
The Mental Body (*Manas*)

You cannot hope to experience inner peace or freedom without understanding the workings of your mind and of human consciousness in general. All behavior, both constructive and destructive, is dependent on our thoughts. By understanding how our thinking works, we discover nothing less than the very secrets of human psychology. With this right perception and understanding of our minds, the door opens to our liberation, as we go through the veil of illusion into the bright day of clarity and wisdom. The study of mind and consciousness, therefore, lies at the heart of yoga.

Obviously mind and consciousness are involved at every level of our being, but because of their subtlety they are considered to reside, as far as yoga's blueprint of humanity is concerned, in the third and fourth sheaths of being. The yogi makes a distinction between the *mental body* (*manomaya kosa*), where the incessant thoughts of human life occur, and the *intellectual body* (*vijnanamaya kosa*), where intelligence and discernment can be found. This chapter deals in detail with the mental body and how the thinking brain, memory, ego, and sensory perception work together, for good or for ill, in our lives. I will introduce the yogic definition of intelligence—making self-aware choices through informed discernment and the exercise of will—but I will return to intelligence and wisdom in the next chapter. It is through this intelligence that we initiate change and free ourselves from ingrained patterns of behavior and steer ourselves incrementally toward illumination and freedom. However, we can hope only to develop intelligence once we understand why we are so often prompted to act without it.

Patanjali, in his *Yoga Sutras*, chose to make the workings of mind and consciousness, both in success and in failure, the central theme of yoga philosophy and practice. In fact, from the yogi's standpoint, practice and philosophy are inseparable. Patanjali's first *sutra* says, "Now I'm going to present the disciplined code of ethical conduct, which is yoga." In other words, yoga is something you *do*. So what do you do? The second *sutra* tells us, "Yoga is the process of stilling the movements and fluctuations of mind that disturb our consciousness." Everything we do in yoga is concerned with achieving this incredibly difficult task. If we achieve it, Patanjali said, the goal and the fruit of yoga will be within our grasp.

My life's work has been to demonstrate that from one's very first *Samasthiti* (standing still and straight) or *Tadasana* (mountain pose) in one's very first class, one is embarking on this task. If one perseveres and refines, gaining strength and clarity, always penetrating from the initial practice, then the techniques of body and breath that yoga offers will lead us to reach the great goal that Patanjali has set. However, a conceptual understanding of what we are trying to do is vital, as long as we do not imagine that it is a substitute for practice. It is an aid to practice. An architectural plan is not the same thing as the building itself, but it is certainly an important element in bringing about its realization.

Yoga has precise definitions of mind and consciousness, and the English words we use do not always correspond well to the Sanskrit. I will explain them as I go along, but suffice to say that normal English usage often uses mind and consciousness synonymously. In the precision of the Sanskrit, mind is described as an aspect or part of consciousness. The mind forms the outer layer of consciousness (*citta*) in the same way as the skeletal and muscular body is the outer sheath that contains the inner body of vital organs and circulatory and respiratory systems. Consciousness means our capacity to be aware, both externally as well as internally, which we call self-awareness. One good image for consciousness is a lake. The pure waters of a lake reflect the beauty around it (external), and one can also see right through the clear water to the bottom (internal). Similarly a pure mind can reflect the beauty in the world around it, and when the mind is still, the beauty of the Self, or soul, is seen reflected in it. But we all know what stagnation and pollution do to a lake. As one has to keep the water of a lake clean, so it is yoga's job to clean and calm the thought waves that disturb our awareness.

What then are the movements and fluctuations of the mind of which Patanjali wrote? In the image of the lake, they are ripples and waves on its surface and currents and movements in its depths. We all recognize how odd thoughts ruffle the surface of our minds, "Oh, I've forgotten to buy the carrots," or "My boss doesn't like me." We notice how outside disturbances create inner ones, "Their mindless chatter is making it impossible for me to concentrate." In yogic terms, mindless chatter, others' or our own, is a lot of distracting ripples. So also do our desires, dislikes, jealousies, doubts, and fears erupt to the surface out of the mind and consciousness. Thoughts arising from memory are considered as a type of wave, as is sleep, or daydreaming. Even ignorance is viewed as a type of movement in consciousness. We will look at these later, but the point here is that a great many forces are constantly troubling the lake, muddying the waters, and agitating the surface. We can see then that restoring our lakes to a state of limpid, crystalline purity and tranquility is a huge undertaking. So we should first look carefully at our consciousness, see what elements combine to make it up, and analyze how they work together.

The Inner Workings of Consciousness

Go into almost any bookshop, and you will see shelf upon shelf of books on self-help, personal problems and growth, psychology, and spiritual practices and paths. What very few of the books get to grips with is the enduring problem at the core of the human dilemma, which is our mind or consciousness—not only, that is to say, the nature of consciousness but above all the way our minds function.

Imagine a manual for a motor car that discusses endlessly and eloquently its bodywork, style, color, acceleration, comfort, and safety features, but that never actually gets down to how an internal combustion engine works. From such a description no one could ever understand, maintain, or mend their cars. Fortunately we can take our cars to the garage where the engines are fully understood and can be repaired. But to whom do we take our own individual minds to get fixed? We can go to a psychologist for advice, but in the end we are eternally obliged to fix our minds ourselves.

Yoga offers us very useful ways to fix the mental problems that cause most of us so much suffering, but first we must understand yoga philosophy's simple description of consciousness. I introduce the word philosophy advisedly here and purposely place it in the same sentence as the word simple. We have the idea that philosophy, which literally means "love of wisdom," has to be complicated, theoretical, and probably incomprehensible to qualify for its name. Yoga philosophy opts for different criteria of excellence; it is straightforward, practical, and most important, applicable *now*.

Yoga identifies three constituent parts to our consciousness (which it calls citta). They are mind (which is called *manas*), ego or self with a small "s" (which is called *ahamkara*), and intelligence (which is called *buddhi*). The mind, as I have said, is the outer layer of consciousness. Its nature is fickleness, unsteadiness, and inability to make productive choices. It cannot decide between good and bad, right or wrong, correct or incorrect. This is the role of the intelligence, which is the inner layer. Ahamkara, or ego, is the innermost layer of consciousness. Literally, ahamkara means "I-shape." It presents itself as our personalities and assumes the identity of the true Self. It is the part of us that hankers after anything that attracts. Whichever layer of consciousness is active expands, causing the others to retract. Yoga describes the relationship between these parts and their relative proportion to each other, and then yoga explains how they react when they encounter the world, which of course they do all the time. Yoga points out how we generally react to the outside world by forming entrenched patterns of behavior that doom us to relive the same events endlessly, though in a superficial variety of forms and combinations. Anyone who looks at history or listens to the litany of woe and war on the daily news will bear this out. Does mankind never learn anything, we ask in exasperation. The historical "change" from killing with stone clubs, to swords, to guns, to nuclear weapons is clearly no change at all, and it's certainly not evolution. The constant is killing, and the choice of means is merely a result of technological inventiveness or "cleverness" at its most self-defeating.

The word cleverness implies a technical facility and dexterity that grows exponentially, whereas intelligence suggests clarity of vision, like pure lake waters that reflect without distortion.

There is nevertheless a chance that we can break free from the imprisoning past and individually train ourselves to control this reactive mechanism in such a way that the old patterns are not repeated; new things truly can happen, and real changes can in fact take place. This dawning clarity is, in essence, the path of yoga.

The evolutionary process I have just described can be summed up individually as "Getting more of what I genuinely desire and less of what I don't." The trick is to recognize which is which and then act on it. The paradox arises in that to train ourselves to achieve this, we have to start by doing a fair bit of what we don't want to do, and rather less of what we think we do. Yoga calls this *tapas*, which I've translated as sustained courageous practice. The French philosopher Descartes said happiness does not consist in acquiring the things we think will make us happy, but in learning to like doing the things we have to do anyway. Try this when you're waiting for a late train or doing the washing up.

If you want to learn how to repair a car, you first need to learn the parts. Similarly, we must now discuss the three components of consciousness and look in detail at the user's manual that yoga offers for the human condition.

Yoga philosophy identifies three main constituents of consciousness, considering them to be an evolution of nature. We all admire the myriad complexities of nature's long evolution—opposable thumbs, the eye of the fish or eagle, the metamorphosis of the frog, a bird's wing, the bat's radar, or at a more subtle level, our own linguistic and grammatical abilities, hard-wired into the brain cells of every healthy human. Yoga asks us to look at the unfolding complexities of consciousness on the evolutionary path that are even more subtle—such as mind, "I-shape," and intelligence—and to question what they are and how they work. Our *mind* processes our thoughts and lived experiences. The *I-shape* allows us to establish a distinction between ourselves and others, whether our mother or the person on the bus next to us. This is perhaps closest to the Western psychological notion of the ego. Beyond this I-shape or ego, and the mental activity of mind, we also have *intelligence* by which we discern and make decisions. Consciousness is composed of these three and is yet greater than the sum of its parts. Let's look more closely at each of them in turn.

Mind: The Human Computer

Mind (manas) in the yogic understanding is both physical and subtle. It covers the entire body, beginning from the brain and nervous systems of the spinal cortex linking outward to the five senses (sight, smell, touch, hearing, and taste), from which it gets most of its information, and then to the five organs of action (hands, feet, tongue, and genital and excretory organs), which it controls and through which it acts. That is why mind is said to be the eleventh sense. Mind is both perceptive and active. The mind is a computer and information storer and sifter, analogous to the central processing unit (CPU) of the computer on your desk. The mind faces out to the external world and deals with the daily affairs of "My knee hurts," "I smell my dinner cooking," "That looks like an interesting film," or "I've forgotten to do my homework." Mind contains the apparatus that makes us outstanding at music, poor at math, handy in the tool room, or gifted at drawing. These qualities are distributed unevenly between people, and though all faculties can be improved upon, no amount of practice will turn an average musician into a Yehudi Menuhin. There is a physical reality to these talents seated in the brain and senses that can be damaged in a physical way, by accidents such as blows to the head, illness, or general deterioration of health through aging or unhealthy living. What mind is and does dies with us. Through mind we engage with, experience, perceive, and interpret the world. Senses perceive, and mind conceives. According to their health and vitality, we enjoy the gift of life to a greater or lesser degree.

Mind is above all clever; clever as they say, as a barrel of monkeys. Like monkeys jumping restlessly from one branch to another, so too the mind flickers from object to object and thought to thought. It is personal, active, outward-looking, and perishable. While the mind is good at sifting and sorting, it is not good at making choices.

Memory, without which we cannot function, is an aspect of mind. The imprints of experiences and sensations are stored by memory within the fabric of consciousness. This permits mind to propose selections such as, "I like the blue, mauve, orange, and pink shirts, but remember that blue suits me best." What we call consumer choice is not a choice but a selection. It offers only an illusion of freedom. The choice to consume has already been made. Mind alone cannot factor in questions like, "Can I afford the shirt?" or "Do I need yet another one?" Mind can select which one to buy but cannot of itself answer the binary problem, "Do I buy a new shirt or don't I?" Mind senses— understands—sight, smell, touch, hearing, and taste, but mind is powerless without its storehouse of past imprints. Therefore when a child is asked to pick up red, he refers to the imprint of red in the cloth of consciousness.

There is a perfectly sensible historical reason for this. Mind, all minds, whether brilliant or dull, are equipped with a simple and instinctual survival tool that is, "Repeat pleasure and avoid pain." This enables us to avoid putting our hands in the fire twice or continually trying to quench our thirst with sea water. The converse of "nasty" implying danger is that "nice" or pleasurable implies the opposite, which is a survival advantage. You can see this most strongly in sexual reproduction. If the sexual act were unpleasant, it would hardly favor the propagation of either our individual genes or the species in general.

If we look at the case of wild animals, we can see this mechanism working, within the context of their lives, almost entirely to their benefit. Think of a brown bear during the autumn salmon run pleasurably guzzling fish after fish. He will need the excess fat to get him through the coming hibernation, and his gluttony, far from being among the seven deadly sins, is an indispensable virtue. But is the context of our lives, alienated from nature as we increasingly are, similar to that of the wild bear? Substitute human for bear and junk food for salmon. Is gluttony likely to prove a winning technique for survival? Not if we all die of clogged arteries at age forty. At the level of the individual, the system that governs the bird, bear, bat, or human brain no longer works so clearly to our advantage as at earlier stages of evolution or in more natural modes of life.

In other words, something programmed in our own brain, which worked very well in the far distant past, is no longer bringing us the benefits it once did. A possible reason for this is contained in the phrase "the context of our lives." Animals are constrained by "short termism." Their actions bear fruit, for good or ill, within short time spans. A gazelle who decided to experiment with junk food would soon end up as a lion's lunch.

In the case of man, the delay between action and consequence, or cause and effect, has gotten longer and longer. No animal has ever planted a field with grain in spring, waited six months for the harvest, and then stored and consumed it over the following year. This is a long span of time. When we tell a child to study hard to pass his exams, we know the consequences might radically alter the quality of his life till his dying day, seventy years later. But what the child is feeling is, "I hate math, I want to watch TV instead." We are back to "nice" and "nasty" and the innate propensity of mind. This is the problem with "long termism," a problem yoga identified more than two thousand years ago. When life's rap on the knuckles is not immediate enough to act as a deterrent, or the reward does not come fast enough to act as a spur, we tend to feel and act like children. We seek immediate gratification.

Take the case of disease. Until recently the greatest danger to health came from such diseases as cholera and typhoid. They operate within a small time scale. Drink contaminated water on Monday, sick on Tuesday, dead on Wednesday. Once the link between water and these diseases was established, we quickly learned through intelligence to purify the water supply. Rapid connections are relatively easy to identify and rectify. If you hit your thumb with a hammer, no one is going to convince you the pain comes from anywhere else. Next time you'll be more careful.

But what of the diseases that plague us now? Are they not degenerative and operative over a very long period? And are not both their avoidance and their cure highly problematic?

We nearly all recognize that there is some connection between the way we live and such illnesses as cancer, heart disease, and arthritis, yet since the process of decline is so gradual and the deadly payoff so long deferred, we find it terribly difficult to make the necessary reforms in our habits of life, even if, at one level, we are actually longing for them.

Take the case of AIDS. I have treated many AIDS patients in my medical class right from the beginning of the epidemic, and so I know the disease and its gradual devastation well. If death supervened the day following our contracting the virus, there would be no AIDS epidemic. Everyone would shun risky or dangerous behavior. But because the onset of sickness is five, ten, fifteen years away, the pull of immediate gratification proves too strong for many people to resist. We find it very hard to change our patterns of behavior, however self-destructive, because of the very nature of the way mind, senses, organs of action, and the external environment work together.

These behavioral ruts seem impossible to jolt ourselves out of, but as we shall presently see, through the understanding of consciousness offered by yoga and the self-mastery gained through its practice, a sustained, progressive reform and change are achievable.

To state that the hereditary bias of mind and senses works often in our disfavor is in no way to condemn this miraculous apparatus that we possess. We must simply come to realize how fast, how powerful, and how tricky it is, impulsive as a wild stallion. The information it gives us—"Fire burns" or "Rice is good to eat"—has proved essential to our survival and still is. Lao Tzu, the Chinese philosopher, said, "Know yourself. Know what is good. Know when to stop." Yoga is concerned to help us reach these goals. Atomic energy is solar fire reproduced on earth. Adequate warmth is desirable. But when we look at the stampede toward the proliferation of nuclear weapons, we must wonder if we have any idea when to stop. A bowl of rice is good. A full belly is desirable. But should it be full twenty-four hours a day? Do we really want "More is better" to be the epitaph of the human race?

In our individual lives, we struggle most with two sorts of action. The first is: Do something "nice" now and at some unspecified time in the future a "nasty" will emerge. Repeat it often enough, and a "nasty" will appear with a compound interest we could well do without. You might call this "From first hangover to cirrhosis." The second is: Do something now that it would be easier not to do (e.g. math homework instead of TV or get up an hour earlier for some *yogasana* practice) and reap the benefit a bit later. Repeat it often enough and harvest the compound interest as the future unrolls. The longer the delay between the primary action/inaction and its secondary effect, the more tempted we are to prevaricate, lie to ourselves, refuse to jump our fences, and take the downhill path. So honesty is a key issue, for without it, "Know yourself" is an impossibility. Thus we deny what is good and never learn when to stop.

Let us now put to one side our mind/brain—gatherer and storer of information and experience and explorer of the world—and examine the second element of consciousness.

I-Shape: The Shape of the Small Self

This is our individual awareness and identification with self, with me, with my singularity and difference from you, my apartness, my feeling in some way of being at the center of everything, and that all that is not me partakes of a degree of otherness. This otherness is not fixed, nor is our I-shape. Indeed, one aspect of the self, which the Sanskrit (ahamkara) conveys, is the constantly changing—ever shrinking and expanding—shape of the self. The great night sky may make us feel small and lonely, but a beautiful sunrise can cause us to feel intimately part of a greater whole, cared for by a benevolent universe. On other occasions the sight of the stars and blackness might bring us to the edge of grasping infinity itself, the source of all our hopes and terrors. So the relationship between self and nonself is fluid. Neither is a fixed quantity. Sometimes we are close and intimate with other people; at other times these same people might seem like our enemies. Yet every time we say the word "I," we feel something hard and monolithic inside us, like a great stone idol.

Whatever the shape of our "I," however defenseless and permeable we allow ourselves to become, a separation between self and other continues to exist in normal consciousness. Even in the rapture of nature's beauty, we know that we are *not* the glowing sunset. There is admiration, not fusion.

Early yoga philosophers identified a grey area between what is me and not me, something that can be either or both, an interface between "I"-ness and the outer world. It is my body. The great attention that yoga, and other practices too, pay to the body derives from its paradoxical position. In death we cannot take it with us, in life we cannot leave it behind. If I cannot take it with me, how can it truly be me? And why therefore should I trouble myself to look after it when in death it betrays me? But if I do not, I begin to decay in life and experience a slow premature death. Yoga calls the body the vehicle of the soul, but as the saying goes, no one ever washes a rented car. Yoga points out that it is in our highest interest to look after this poor conveyance, at every level, from health to mind to self to soul. The conundrum of body is the starting point in yoga from which to unravel the mystery of human existence.

What is the point of having an individual I-shape? Could we, as with our appendix, live without it? Why is this evolutionary trait present to a greater or lesser extent in the whole animal kingdom? Why most of all in human beings?

The most natural answer is simply that singularity of body requires singularity of awareness. Imagine a car with two independent steering wheels and two drivers. It would never stay on the road. Self locomotion necessitates a single "I" awareness linked through mind, senses, and body to the environment that provides food, air, and water. Since each biological entity is subtly or grossly different, and recognizes that in itself, so it needs to recognize difference in others. At the most basic level, sexual reproduction demands we differentiate between male and female. Wind pollination does not. No two grains of sand may be the same, but as they do not move about of their own volition, forage for food, or reproduce, the last thing they need is a highly developed ego.

I have said that our I-shape is fluid. When we throw ourselves into a great ideal or cause, or even go along as fans to support our national sports team at the Olympics, we are subsumed in a larger identity, for the moment laying aside the burden of the individual self. But this collectivity is both partial and temporary. This is still I-consciousness. It is at best a poor substitute for primal unity.

Our "I-ness" is an identifier. We need to identify with a certain particularity in order to maintain biological and mental integrity. All this is to the good, so how is it that the words ego and egoistic carry such negative connotations?

It is because the surface of our I-shape is covered with super glue. Memories, possessions, desires, experiences, attachments, achievements, opinions, and prejudices stick to the "I" like barnacles to the hull of a ship. The I-shape's contact with the outer world is through mind and senses. All the treasure and glory and misery of that contact are passed back to ego, which accumulates them and declares, "This totality is me." My success, my wife, my car, my job, my woes, my wants, my, my, my. And the pure single identity succumbs to the disease of elephantiasis, in which our self becomes grossly enlarged, coarsened, and thickened.

In India there is a lovely name for girls—Asmita. It means "I-ness." *Aham* means "I." *Asmi* means "am." This I-am-ness is *asmita. Aham* means I and *akara* means shape. When I identify myself with my possessions and attributes, it is *ahamkara*. From this derives "me, my, mine." When I identify myself with "I", that is *asmita*—"I-ness." It reflects the beauty of the gift of singularity and uniqueness that all who live possess. It also, however, means pride. You can see the connection—overweening pride is the symptom of the diseased self. Our bodies can fall sick, likewise our minds. So also the self. The answer to our earlier question as to why mankind is so prone to this engorgement of the ego lies probably in our extraordinary mental capacities for speech and memory. Communication and memory permit the ego to feed incessantly off the experiences relayed to it by mind. Naturally it puts on weight and falls sick.

A long time ago, yogis examined this unsatisfactory state of affairs. They saw how the bias in mind of "repeat pleasure, avoid pain" for all its survival usefulness could lead to trouble. Where was the problem with "I-consciousness"? The benefit is clear—single awareness in a single biological entity. Is it possible, they asked, that the singularity of awareness, the I-ness, is not the same thing as my true Self, the essence of my being, but merely for practical day-to-day purposes impersonates it and, as it were, by force of habit has actually come to believe in that impersonation?

That is the nub of it. Ego has been compared to the filament in a light bulb, which, because it glows with light, proclaims itself to be the light's source, electricity. In reality the light that shines from I-consciousness devolves from another and deeper source, one unknowable in daily life, but which mankind has always intuitively felt to exist. We connect it to our beginnings, to an original oneness out of which we have emerged. We connect it to our destination, to an ultimate whole to which we shall one day return. We connect it to the sky, our invisible gateway to infinity. What we cannot achieve, living as we do in a world of multiplicity, diversity, difference, and separation, of "getting and spending" as the poet says, is to perceive that source and ultimate unity within ourselves, and in the complexities of everyday living. We can perhaps sense its presence and dimly half remember it like the face of a long lost love or timidly apprehend it like the face of the lover we yearn for but have yet to meet.

The most common word we give to this is soul. If the "I" attaches itself to consciousness, it becomes ego (ahamkara). If the "I" can be erased, awareness of soul infuses the consciousness. This is not the true realization of the soul. The soul is a separate entity and should not be confused with any form of "I" consciousness. Nevertheless, when ego is quiescent, consciousness senses the reality of the soul, and the light of soul expresses itself through the translucent consciousness.

To an extent, we all sense the presence of soul in our origin and our end. Looking at the world around us, we are torn between feelings that "soul cannot be in this" and yet, "if soul exists at all, it must be in this also." We guess it to be unlimited by our notions of space and time. Its existence is not defined by or confined to the span of our years between the cradle and the grave. Those brief years are the province of the I-shape of consciousness, which is born, grows, flourishes, withers, and dies in the body that bears it. It is democratic: if in us then equally in others. It is not personal; if anything, it is we who belong to it.

If we mistake this separate, necessary but temporary "I-awareness" for our true and abiding identity, if we confuse it with soul, we are in a cleft stick. What we all most desire is to live and to be a part of life. By choosing to identify with a part of ourselves that MUST die, we condemn ourselves to death. By embracing a false identity, accepting the confusion at face value, man places himself in a position of almost unbearable tension. Yoga calls this state "ignorance" and sees it as our fundamental affliction, the matrix of error from which all other misperceptions and errors flow. From our ignorant identification with our ego and its mortality arises man's creativity and his destructiveness, the glory of culture, the horror of his history.

We embark on great and wonderful projects to affirm that the egoic self will not die. What are the pyramids of Egypt but an attempt to cheat death? They are a marvel of organization, engineering, geometry, and astronomy, but the motivating force behind them was the Pharaohs' lust for personal immortality and vanity in believing there was a means for his human, kingly ego to cheat the grave.

A voice within us always whispers that this is a forlorn hope, yet still in innumerable ways we endeavor to perpetuate a part of ourselves whose days are numbered, or to comfort ourselves in advance for the coming loss. What is the attraction of great luxury except this? Consumerism cannot be the gateway to immortality. It is an ineffective and temporary balm against mortality.

To endure the fears of impermanence and to struggle against the inevitable is a tiring business, so at the same time we long equally for loss of self, for fusion, for submergence and transcendence, for release from the burden of ego. The egoic self is an exhausting traveling companion, forever demanding that his caprices be pandered to, that his whims be obeyed (though he is never satisfied), and his fears be calmed (though they never can be).

The lovely *Asmita*, single awareness in single body, is thus transformed into an insatiable, paranoid, vainglorious tyrant, although this is a phenomenon we normally notice more easily in other people.

The reason for this sad transformation is ignorance, the misperception whereby a part of us is taken for the whole. Much of yoga practice and ethic is concerned with cutting the ego down to size and removing the veil of unknowing that obscures its vision. This can be done only with the intervention and assistance of the third constituent of consciousness.

Intelligence: The Source of Discernment

This is intelligence (buddhi). Yoga, once again, makes an important distinction between intelligence and mind (manas). The specific quality of mind is cleverness. All people are clever compared to other forms of life. Yoga states clearly that it is not the fact of being less clever than your neighbor that makes you stupid. Stupidity is the absence of intelligence. Stupidity can be behaving in a certain way or not learning from our mistakes. We are all stupid sometimes. Relatively speaking we are all clever all the time. A rocket scientist or professor of linguistics may be more stupid than a peasant in the fields or a worker in a factory. He may well be much cleverer but that does not necessarily make him more intelligent. Let me give you an example. Scientifically advanced nations invent many complex and terrible weapons. To do this they must be clever. Then they sell these weapons indiscriminately around the world, and the arms end up in the hands of their enemies. Is this clever or stupid? If stupid, did their stupidity consist of a sudden loss of cleverness or of an absence of intelligence? Mind is certainly highly inventive. But is that the same as being innovative? To innovate is to introduce the new, to engage in a process of change. To invent is to produce a different variation of the old. This is a subtle and important distinction, for we often mix the two up. For example, if someone always makes me angry, I may express my anger in a thousand different ways, inventing new words or actions to do so. The day I choose not to respond with anger, something new has taken place. This is innovation. There is change. Yoga tries to help us to truly innovate, to develop the intelligence that allows us to create a new relationship to our ego and our world. This new relationship is dependent on perceiving the world objectively and truthfully and on making choices, discerning what is best.

Intelligence has two overriding characteristics. First, it is reflexive; it can stand outside the self and perceive objectively, not just subjectively. When I am being subjective, I say I hate my job. When I am being objective, I say I have the skills to get a better job. This first quality makes possible intelligence's second. It can choose. It can choose to perform an action that is new, that is innovative. It can initiate change. It can decide to jump out of the ruts in which we are all stuck and strike out on a path for its own evolution. Intelligence does not chat. It is the quiet, determined, clear-eyed revolutionary of our consciousness. Intelligence is the silent or sleeping partner in consciousness, but when it awakes it is the senior or dominant partner.

If we glance back at mind (manas) and I-shape (ahamkara), the two conservative stalwarts of consciousness, we will see that logically they are governed by mechanisms that resist change. Mind and the senses that inform it seek to repeat pleasure and avoid pain. We have seen the rationale behind this but at the same time must admit that it is essentially a holding pattern of behavior, rooted in the experience of the past. It is in consequence likely to shy away from innovation and thus stifle the possibility of evolution. We saw that I-shape or ego defines itself as the totality of the experiences that have accrued to it in the past: my childhood, my university degree, my bank account. I-Shape, or Ego, is the running total of all that has happened up until now. It is in love with the past. Why? What does ego fear most? Its own death. Where is that? In the future. So of course ego is happiest with endless variations on the past. It is comfortable rearranging the same old furniture in the same old room and standing back and saying, "Doesn't it look different?" Does it? Yes. Is it? No. What ego does not want to do is throw away the furniture and leave the room. That is the unknown. The unknown resuscitates all its panic fears of its own impermanence, the fear that one day its impersonation of the true self, the unknown soul, will be unmasked, at which point its existence, as it has hitherto known it, will terminate.

Early European travelers in India were often horrified to discover that the goal of religious practice was an end to the illusion of the lasting reality of the egoic self. They reacted to this as a sort of living suicide. Paradoxically they also respected it. Experience of *samadhi* reveals to us that ego is not the source of Self. We transcend ego identification. After samadhi we return to our ego but use it as a necessary tool for living, not a substitute for soul. Ego no longer limits us with its pettiness, fears, or cravings.

The Sanskrit word for philosophy, *darsan*, means vision or sight. This is the sight of ourselves, an objective vision, acting as a mirror to the self. This is the reflexive quality of intelligence. Plato said that it is not enough to know (which is subjective): We must know that we know. This is objective. It is the consciousness of being conscious that makes us human. Trees are conscious too; a clump of oaks harmoniously spreads its limbs for the benefit of each leaf, each individual tree in the group. But they are not consciously conscious. The consciousness of nature is unconscious. The history of humankind can be described as a journey from unconsciousness to conscious consciousness or self-awareness. If this is correct, then it must operate at the level of the individual, and of the species, as consciousness is permeable.

What is the advantage conferred by the mirror of intelligence? Simply that we can see ourselves as if from a distance. Suddenly the egoic self becomes an object. Normally it is the subject, incapable of seeing things except from its own point of view. A real mirror permits us to see ourselves as if from outside, therefore to notice what we could not otherwise see, food stains on our ties for example. Thus we can make changes in our appearances if we are disturbed by the images we see. In fact, consciousness is a double mirror, able to reflect the objects of the world, or the soul within.

We can choose to take off and clean our tie. We can choose to start asana practice and cleanse our bodies. "We can choose." That is the second aspect of intelligence. Based on objective information, we can choose to clean our ties or not to clean them. We can start asana practice or sleep longer in the morning. In Latin, intelligence means "to choose between." It does not mean simply to think.

Have you ever noticed that when we have a problem we say, "Shh! Wait, let me think"? But what we really mean is "Shh! Wait, let me stop thinking." We want to see clearly, and so we need to freeze-frame the incessant flow of pulsating images, words, and their subliminal associations that are erupting from mind. Mind produces thought and image all the time, like a television with no off switch. Thought moves too fast to catch and never, of its own accord, stops. It is an unending analogue wave flowing from our brains out into the ether. It cannot re-form itself. Thought cannot solve the problems caused by thought any more than a faulty engine can mend itself without the objective view and intervention of the mechanic. That is the role of intelligence: to stop, to discern, to discriminate, to intervene.

Intelligence performs its task firstly by its ability to freeze-frame the flow of thought. This is what we call cognition. Cognition is the process of knowing and includes both awareness and judgment. Cognition allows us to perceive *in the present moment* that at the heart of a situation is a choice. With the image of thought no longer flickering, we see ourselves objectively in a position where we can ask, "Do I now do this or do I now do that?" Time pauses in a moment of awareness and reflection in which suddenly our destiny is ours to command. "Do I eat a second scoop of ice cream or do I stop now?" The choice may be hard, but at least it is simple. We find ourselves at a parting of the ways that, however trivial in itself, is somehow momentous to us.

Imagine you wake up early one morning and ask yourself, "Shall I get up and do a bit of yogasana practice for once or shall I turn over and sleep for another hour?" In a way we desire both, but recognize that this is impossible. There is a choice, a fork in the road before us. Both paths have their attractions, but obviously one is easier than the other. Our cognitive intelligence has brought us to a clear perception of choice, but at the moment of decision we are still stuck. Is the harder path (getting out of bed) really an option?

Thanks to the second aspect of intelligence, yes, it is. This is the property of will, or volition. This will is sometimes called "conation," which is why we say in yoga that intelligence is both "conative" and "cognitive." Will is what gets our feet out of bed and translates our awareness of choice into action. Will is what converts the harder option from hypothesis into reality. I have often described Hatha Yoga as the Yoga of Will.

Now you are out of bed. The battle is won but not the war. Would it not be nice now to make a coffee and read the morning paper for an hour? Getting up was an achievement, a step in the right direction . . . but was it enough? Another moment of cognition, of choice, of the exercise of will. Soon you are doing yoga practice at 6.30 a.m. This is new, a first, an initiation, an innovation.

This is history being made, your personal history, thanks to the mirror and scissors of intelligence—see, choose, act. Afterward you will probably measure the benefit of the practice in terms of physical well-being as you set off for work, a certain vitality, and some satisfaction at your own activity and self-discipline. What you have also exercised, along with the components of body, is that too-often dormant component of consciousness, intelligence itself.

And tomorrow, when the alarm clock rings, it is all to do again. Or perhaps not quite all. If a well-toned body works better each day, surely the same is true for a well-honed intelligence. For our bodies, the fruit of our sustained, intelligent effort will be, in its widest sense, health. But at another level, what we are really gaining, (and this is the cause of our satisfaction) is self-control.

This is a point of huge significance. Logically, with health and self-control, we are increasingly able to direct our lives. We feel happy when we are directing our own lives because we are experiencing a growing freedom. We are exploring the possibilities of life on earth through the release and realization of our own potential. Freedom is the innermost desire of all our hearts. It is the only desire that leads us toward unity and not separation. It makes possible our aspirations to love and be loved, and on its farthest shore, touches that union with infinity that is the ground and the goal of yoga. If infinity seems a long way off, let us not forget that when, by an act of effortful intelligence, we remove our feet from the warm bed to the cold floor, we have taken our first step.

By now we have made a quick tour of mind, ego, and intelligence, which together form consciousness. There is much more to be said, and more, with this model as a guide, which you can discover for yourself. Consciousness is greater than the sum of its parts, and I will talk about this later. I have mentioned some of the defects inherent in mind and small-self (I-consciousness), but not yet those of intelligence. Our first job is to awaken and vitalize intelligence before we look at what can go wrong. (Patanjali called it *sattva-suddhi*—purity or cleansing of the intelligence.)

Now I want to describe how mind (and the senses that inform it), ego, and intelligence collaborate (or not) in a trivial everyday situation. We have the model in our mind's eye of consciousness as a circle divided into three intercommunicating segments. This is static, which the world certainly is not, so we shall launch a challenge to consciousness in the form of an external sense object. This will be a very large tub of vanilla ice cream.

You have arrived home late and tired from work. On the way you stopped off for a pizza and so are no longer particularly hungry. Once in the kitchen, as if by magic, you find yourself opening the freezer door. Inside sits a tub of vanilla ice cream.

The following sequence of events takes place:

1. Your eyes (sense organs) light on the ice cream, read the label (vanilla), and carry the information back to mind for decoding and

identification. A link is established: a) external object, b) sense organ, c) mind.

2. Mind (as it always does) relays this information to the egoic self. The links of the chain are now a) + b) + c) + d) ego.

3. Quick as a flash, ego and mind go into a huddle, and memory, which is contained in mind, is brought into play. A question is automatically put to memory, "Does the act of eating vanilla ice cream result in pleasure or pain?"

4. Without hesitation memory replies, "Pleasure."

5. Ego says "OK, give it to me." And mind coordinates the hand (organ of action) movements necessary to take the tub off the shelf, open it, and find a spoon. The rest is history.

Let us now go back to stage 4 and see if any other outcome might have been possible and, if so, how.

5a) Mind and ego are vaguely aware of a sort of static buzz in the background of consciousness, as if someone were trying to get their attention. This makes them uneasy, so they turn round (away from the open fridge) and see intelligence jumping up and down. "May I ask memory a question?" it asks.

6a) Mind and self shuffle their feet, sensing trouble, but finally reply, "We'd rather you didn't, but if you insist we cannot deny you a chance."

7a) "Thank you," says intelligence. "Memory, please tell me what happens when you eat ice cream, night after night? What are the *consequences?*"

8a) Memory has a truthful nature though on occasion it can make mistakes. Memory replies, "You put on a lot of weight, can't fit into your new trousers, have sinusitis, and your arthritis flares up." Left to itself, memory from past acquired taste will make the mistake of saying, "Go ahead—eat, enjoy." It is the intervention of intelligence that poses the more complex question, "Do we live to eat, or eat to live?"

9a) Intelligence continues to hold the floor. "Let me summarize our predicament," it says. "We all enjoy eating ice cream, even in excess. We all hate the secondary consequences of this, you especially, ego, being so vain about your figure. It seems to me we have a choice—to eat it or not to eat it. That must be clear to us all." (Cognition + choice)

10a) Poor mind is utterly confused, as, in spite of its name, it does not really have a mind of its own. It will run in any direction, like a dog after a ball. Normally it lets ego give the orders, and ego is now very upset. "I *always* eat ice cream when I'm tired after a long, hard day. It's a great comfort to me. I owe it to myself. It's who I am."

11a) Intelligence, (who is also annoyed about the trousers, though in its case it is more about the stupid waste of money) speaks up for the last time. "For once I'm going to put my foot down (Will). I'm fed up with the rut you two are in, always the same, day in, day out, and then whining about the consequences, or dreaming about how good things used to be or will be again one day. Nothing's going to change unless we do (Challenge). Mind, please tell hand to move away from the ice cream and shut the freezer door." Which it does.

12a) And next day they all felt better for the way things had turned out. In fact ego was very smug and had quite persuaded itself that leaving the ice cream had been its idea all along.

If we can train ourselves to compress all the steps from 1a to 12a in this little story into a second and then we use them dozens of times a day in every situation, then we will have a disciplined mind, a pliant (i.e. not rigid) ego, an acute vibrant intelligence and, as a result, a smoothly functioning, integrated consciousness. You may have noticed that the example of getting out of bed to practice yogasana concerned embracing a positive, whereas the matter of the ice cream involved avoiding a negative. In either case, intelligence operates in the same manner. It is like a rudder on a boat that must be able to steer both to port and starboard. If not, the craft would turn in circles.

Nevertheless, when trying to alter embedded behavioral patterns, it is preferable to create a positive formulation. "Let me find out the right way to lift my chest," is better than "Let me not get it wrong again." We see this with children. "Don't stand there," is an order that only serves to tell the child he or she is doing something wrong. The unconscious mind, relatively more powerful in the young, cannot work out from this where is the right place to stand. Only the rational conscious mind can do that. "Come and stand over here," is an instruction that makes full sense to the child. Otherwise he or she will live in dread of doing wrong rather than the hope and expectation of doing right. Since ingrained patterns of behavior, which yoga calls *samskara* or subliminal impressions, lie, as the word subliminal suggests, largely in our unconscious, it is in our own interests to emphasize the new and positive action and not dwell on the negative past. Before we can strike on this new path, we must understand how these ingrained habits and patterns of behavior or conditioned reflexes—samskara—so often control us.

Samskara: Freeing Yourself from Habit

If consciousness is like a lake, there are primary waves or fluctuations of consciousness on the surface of the lake. These are easily discernible. An example is that if you are invited to dinner by dear friends and, at the last minute, they ring to cancel, then you're very disappointed. That is a primary wave on the surface of the lake. You're disappointed, you're unhappy, you feel let down, and you deal with that on the surface. You have to calm yourself down, get over your disappointment.

That is a challenge, an external challenge as it were, that causes a ripple on the surface.

The secondary fluctuations or waves are different. Those are the ones that rise up from the bottom of the lake. The bottom of a lake is covered in sand and so, if in life you experience a sufficient number of disappointments, the ripple on the surface creates a wave that goes down to the bottom, and imperceptibly that ripple creates a little bank in the sand, so there is a little mound of disappointment. As a result you will find yourself frequently disappointed or sad as this mound at the bottom sends off secondary fluctuations or waves.

Let us look at another common example. If you constantly find yourself being irritable, annoyed by something—your wife, your children, your parents, or anything at all—a sufficient number of irritable reactions will create, imperceptibly, not in one time only, a little mound of irritability at the bottom of the lake of consciousness, and that will eventually make you what we call an irritable person, an angry person. If you have smoked since you were sixteen, every time you pick up a cigarette in the day you are also brainwashing yourself. "In this situation I pick up a cigarette" sends a little ripple down through consciousness that adds to the "take a cigarette" mound. That's why cigarettes are more difficult than almost anything else to give up. Aside from their physical cravings, we create mental cravings because the habit is very repetitive. The habit of smoking puts itself into every situation. The triggers to that situation are so many that many smokers still sometimes want to smoke even years after they have stopped because the mound is still there.

When you have an anger, irritability, or disappointment mound, the conditioned reflex works like this: Suppose you're irritable with your parents, and your mother comes into the room. She might only say "Dinner's ready," but the irritability reflex is ready to spring up. She has said nothing to irritate you, but the irritability mound means that any incoming stimulus connected to her sends a wave down through the lake and hits the irritability mound. So we get a distorted and secondary wave of bad-tempered thought bouncing up from the floor of the lake. The accumulated predisposition to bad temper rears up and says, "Oh, it's my mother; she's so irritating," and even though she only announced dinner, you reply, "Oh, alright, I'm coming, I'm coming." There's an irritation in the response that isn't warranted. This often happens between husband and wife. The same predisposition occurs whether you are talking about a smoking habit or about accumulated disappointment. Somebody who has encountered a great deal of disappointment, who has got that mound, in any situation, is likely to feel predisposed to disappointment. When something happens, they don't say, "Oh, this could be good," or "Let's see how this turns out." They say, "Oh, dear, I don't know, this is going to go wrong." That's the disappointment wave sending off a secondary reflex thought of unjustified negativity.

As these things are built up over time, they can be removed only over time. It's not because you give up smoking for a day or you guard your tongue and don't snap at your wife for a day or you say, "Yes I'll look on the bright side of life," that you remove the mound at the bottom of the lake that has been built up over probably many years or even your whole life. By now, it's a big mound, sending out powerful waves that are nevertheless difficult to detect.

The practice of yoga is about reducing the size of the subliminal mounds and setting us free from these and other fluctuations or waves in our consciousness. Everybody aspires to be free. No one wants to be manipulated by unseen forces, but effectively, the banks of samskara in the dark depths of the unconscious do just that. As stimuli from the conscious surface travel rapidly down through the levels of the lake, they encounter uncharted banks of sediment that cause secondary waves of thought. These in turn stimulate, in a way that is beyond our comprehension or control, behavior that is both reactive and inappropriate. Our reactions are preconditioned and therefore unfree. We cannot break out of the old pattern of behavior, however much we long to. In the end, we may accept the situation and just say, "It's the way I am," "Life always lets me down," "Things just make me so angry," or "I have an addictive personality."

If you don't smoke for one day, you actually take away from the smoking sandbank at the bottom of the lake so the sandbank is fractionally smaller. But the second day you don't smoke, you still want to smoke because you've got a one-day "I don't smoke" mound and a twenty-four-year "I do smoke mound." Obviously it is through the continued practice of creating "I don't smoke," "I'm not disappointed," or "I don't get irritable" mounds that, little by little, we re-form ourselves. We diminish the size of the negative mounds and turn them into positive samskara such as "I am a nonsmoker," "I am good-natured," or "I am equable." Then you build up banks of good nature, bonhomie, openness, nonsmoking, or whatever you want. These form a good character, and they make our lives much easier. Somebody with good habits of life is an agreeable person able to make his way in life. This is a reward from practice, cleanliness, contentment, and from a process of self-reform that you can undertake even without yoga. Yoga is a support to it obviously, yoga is a way to it, but that doesn't mean there is no reform of samskara outside of yoga. However, yoga is a powerful tool for liberating ourselves from unwanted, ingrained patterns. Through it, we identify, acknowledge, and progressively change them. What is unique to yoga is an ability to take us further, to an unconditioned freedom, because yoga sees even good habits as a form of conditioning or limitation.

Yoga never forgets that the end purpose is not just to remove bad samskara. We also have to cultivate good deeds to build up good samskara. Of course we first have to weed out the bad. But the yogic compass always returns to the notion of emancipation. So what we want is for the bottom of the lake to be flat so that we don't get any secondary fluctuations bouncing off the bottom. That is freedom. But practically speaking, you can't go from bad samskara in one jump to freedom. You've got to go from bad samskara to good samskara to freedom. It's a logical progression. It's doable. Theoretically you could go from bad to total redemption, and there may be cases where this happens, but it would be very rare.

In practical terms, most of us have built up negative habits. You want to turn them into positive habits and then into no habits. As progress reaches into the subtle levels of *kosa*, you don't avoid smoking because you are "a nonsmoker" or because smoking is bad. You are not invoking a duality of good versus bad. Similarly, you do not have to bite off your tongue to avoid giving an angry retort to people who irritate you; you're not being self-consciously good. It simply becomes second nature to be free. You might give an angry answer to a rude person, you might give a courteous answer to a rude person, but either way you act in freedom, you act appropriately, unconditioned by the past.

In teaching it is sometimes necessary for me to act the role of anger. I have to appear "mercilessly merciful" in order to save students from themselves. The anger response is appropriate. But I am not attached to the anger. The anger role does not disturb the bottom of the lake and create a pattern. As soon as I turn away from the student, I put down the anger. I am detached and ready to deal with the next student with friendliness or humor, or whatever is appropriate to his or her needs. I do not get caught up, yet I can engage fully in the comedy and tragedy of the human drama.

Suppose you've always eaten too much chocolate, then you give it up for a long time and free yourself from chocolate. Later on, if someone offers you some chocolate, you can actually say "Yes" or "No" to the chocolate, but you know that if you pick up a piece of chocolate and eat one piece, you won't have to buy the whole chocolate shop to satisfy a craving that is still dormant within you. You can touch it lightly and say, "Great, that's enough," but you're not caught.

So you're acting in freedom. That gives you moderation and lightness, and you're dealing with the situation as it is. You're not a prisoner of past badness or past goodness. This has significant karmic implications.

Everybody wants to have what is called good karma rather than bad, so we're trying to make karmic consequences less unpleasant. Pleasant effects derive from positive samskara. So build these up, and you get good consequences. This makes life pleasant, livable, and agreeable, for us and for others. There is a real social benefit. But the yogic goal is freedom so the yogi says, "I want to be free of consequence; I want to be free of karmic causality. Let me act in the present, unconditioned even by the good imprints bringing good results. I will try to cultivate actions so that they are reaction free." He will not be tied either to the past or, through self-interested motivation, to the future. He will simply act cleanly in the present. If we understand the relationship between samskara and *karma*, of actions and their consequences, we can break the chain of causality. The advantage of sustained and dedicated practice over time (tapas) is that it creates lasting results. What we do over time removes what we have created over time. We cannot leap to freedom in one bound or one immersion in a holy river. This is a dream, an illusion. Resurfacing ego will always grab us back. The immersion is a beginning and a declaration of good intent. We wash away our stains and heal our wounds and frailties over many minutes, in many hours, in many years of sustained, mindful application. Nevertheless even beginners can move rapidly from debit to credit, and the quality of life can change significantly for the better. Presence of mind, self-control, and creative direction embrace us, and we gain the strength to persevere in the face of remaining adversities.

Whether one agrees with the technicalities of karmic causality or not, everyone desires progressively to raise the threshold of their intelligence and to reap the benefits. This is a sort of karmic moving staircase, an impulse toward moving up and fear of the consequences of moving down. We must be careful, however, that the idea of progress does not project us into a future that never comes.

The point we are seeking to reach is where we can act directly in the present. Direct action stems from direct perception, the ability to see reality in the present, as it is, without prejudice, and act accordingly. This is what it truly means to live in the present moment. If we perceive and act in the present, then we are coming closer to the yogic ideal of what is called an action without taint or without color. Actions are either black, which means they are entirely rooted in selfish motivations and lead to painful consequences, or white, disinterested and good or, like most actions, grey, in that they stem from mixed motives and therefore bring mixed results. That's the normal way of the world. The yogic action is an action that is absolutely unfettered by past habit and without desire for personal reward in the future. It is the right thing in this present moment just because it is right and is colorless or taint-free. Its great benefit is that you can act in the world without creating reaction. The benefit of that for a yogi, in relation to freedom, is that he is trying to free himself from the karmic wheel of becoming. The yogi wants to get off the merry-go-round of cause and effect.

He knows that pleasure leads to pain and pain to pleasure in an endless cycle. It is an exhilarating ride, and the goal for most people is to eliminate the pain and experience only pleasure. The yogi knows this is impossible and takes the radical solution of transcending the endless chain of causality. He does not cease to engage in life, on the contrary, but he can act without being tainted. That is why we say his actions are without taint or color, and it is only possible when the ego that rides on the merry-go-round ceases to impersonate the Soul. The Soul is always outside the game of life, a Seer, not a player, and so when the ego-based human consciousness loses its identity in the Soul it can no longer be ensnared in pains and pleasures. The ego is then understood to be no more than an actor's mask for the true Self.

Few people have ever reached this level of detachment. Humanity lives for the most part in grey actions, with mixed results, but nurtures an ethical resolve gradually to shift from grey to white. What impedes this self-reforming process is that we have little awareness, let alone control, of the waves of thought that arise in the depths of the unconscious. Few of us possess the clarity and dexterity to catch the currents that arise from ingrained habits and conditioned reflexes. Yet if we understood the complex role of memory, we are more likely to use it skillfully and act with greater awareness and freedom.

Memory: Liberation or Bondage

When Pavlov rang his bell for the dogs at mealtimes, the dogs salivated because the bell hit a "bell equals mealtime" mechanism in them associating with and triggering memory. The bell triggered the "time to eat" response, and salivation occurred instantly. The dogs didn't say, "Wait a minute, this is a secondary wave. This is only a bell." It is very difficult for us to pick up the secondary wave rising from the unconscious toward the surface. We are caught up in the action that it provokes, both like salivation, at a physical and sensorial level or the level of doing something (salivating is an action). We're caught up in the consequence before we can interrupt it.

For example, sex or violence in films acts like this on us. Even if we dislike or disapprove of them at a conscious level, they create secondary waves from unconscious sexual or aggression sandbanks that muddy the waters of consciousness. Only someone who is completely free of causality is beyond the dangers of pollution. The advertising business is largely based on the trick of triggering a response in the customer's unconscious mind. Our consciousness increasingly becomes what we feed it.

It's very difficult to be aware of these secondary waves rising. We always think that we are reacting in a certain situation to the primary stimulus, the ruffle on the surface of consciousness, but in fact, far more than we can ever realize, we are reacting to the predisposition that is in the samskara at the bottom of the lake. Consumers buy products without knowing what it is that has unconsciously motivated them to do so. We think we're acting in freedom; we convince ourselves that we are, but in reality we are manipulated or influenced by these waves. The word influence comes from the Latin "to flow in," which shows that their language understood thought as a current or wave. The yogi wants to see and act directly so he needs a flat-bottomed lake in order to act solely in response to the stimulus that comes from outside and that is on the surface.

How do we catch secondary waves coming up from the floor of consciousness? Let us say you are driving a car and a small absent-mindedness or selfishness on the part of another driver releases a wave of anger in you. Before you know it, you are honking your horn, cursing, and driving aggressively yourself. Does it do any good? Do you feel better for letting your serenity be so easily shattered? Does blaming the other driver restore your peace of mind? No.

If you want to intercept the secondary waves rising, you need speed and clarity of perception, an acute self-awareness. If your lake is muddy and impure, if there are lots of toxins in your system clouding your vision, clarity of vision is impossible. If your liver is sluggish with toxins, your brain will be impaired because the liver is not filtering the blood. Your nervous system will be slow to react to danger, but disproportionate in the degree of stress it registers. To gain health, you have to know the unconscious mind, which expresses itself within the nervous system. If the nerves are disturbed, you feel the weakness of the mind. As long as the nerves are strong, stable, and elastic, the mind is stable. When mind is stable, the sediment held in suspension that clouds it sinks to the bottom, and the consciousness becomes limpid.

Cleanliness and contentment are bound together. As we shall see, they are the first two ethical injunctions of *niyama* concerning our behavior toward ourselves. As yoga practice cleans the system and rests the nerves, clarity, contentment, and serenity establish themselves. Contentment means the thought waves in the lake of consciousness are less turbulent. You are starting to bring about Patanjali's statement, "Yoga is about stilling the turbulence of consciousness."

Someone who is clouded, toxic, sluggish, discontented (blaming others is a prime cause of discontent), and restive in mind is never going to catch a secondary wave coming to the surface. It will have expressed itself in action before they even notice it. It is through the acute awareness and speed of action that we cultivate in asana and *pranayama* that we can reform ourselves. In addition, by breathing before acting, we are able to slow down our responses, inhale divinity, and surrender ego in our exhalation. This momentary pause allows us the time for cognitive reflection, corrective reaction, and reappraisal. It is the momentary pause in the process of cause and effect that allows us to begin the process of freedom.

The endless process is breath, cognitive reflection, corrective reaction, reappraisal, and action. Eventually this process blends together in such a manner that we discover we have pulled ourselves into the present moment, no past, no future, but action and right perception soldered together in a peerless moment, and then another moment and another. Eventually, we are no longer caught up in the movement of time as a sequence or current sweeping us along, but we experience it as a series of discrete and present moments. No rising thought wave can escape the sharpness of such vision. It is what we call presence of mind. Great sportsmen possess it at the level of the body's intelligence. They seem to have so much more time to act than other players. It is as if the game slows down around them, and they can dominate it as they please.

Asana and pranayama teach us how unsolicited thought throws us off balance. Take the standing pose *Ardha Chandrasana* (half-moon asana), balancing on one leg, the other horizontal, arm extended upward. We get the balance, but the moment the thought arises, "Oh, wonderful, I'm doing it!" we wobble or topple. Only in stillness of mind can it be successfully maintained. Similarly in pranayama, we see how breath and consciousness interact. A disturbance or irregularity in one creates its counterpart in the other. When breath is calmed and attention focused on its inward movement, then consciousness is no longer jerked by outer stimuli. Similarly, if the consciousness is steady and stable, the breath moves with rhythm. Either way it is receptive and passive, no more hungrily seeking distraction or entertainment. This frees it to let its attention gravitate toward the most profound level of consciousness in the depths of the lake. Normally this level appears as our unconscious as no light of awareness penetrates it. But if the lake is clear, no rising wave can catch us by surprise. There is no mystery here. It is about training, self-education. If we learn reflection and correction in equipoise, where any movement or alteration is detectable and its source revealed, then we have acquired the sensitivity that brings self-knowledge—the threshold of wisdom. We know when we are reacting to an external challenge in a straightforward manner, or when the hidden sandbanks of previous conditioning are trying to influence and warp our response. We can now identify thought as a deliberative, useful, and necessary process, a great gift and talent apart from thought as meaningless disturbance, mindless chatter, a radio we cannot switch off, and also from thought as a subtle form of interference from the past, a self-sabotaging mechanism lodged in our unconscious memory.

We have looked at the process of turning negative habits into positive ones as a prelude to the larger freedom of unalloyed moment-to-moment perception and wisdom, but one might legitimately ask this question. "What happens if a negative sandbank has been created in unconscious memory by a single past event such as a traumatic accident ten years ago, the spontaneous recall of which may continue to trouble the present as latent, hidden impressions resurface." There is no countervailing positive sandbank we can build up, and so we would seem to be imprisoned by an unchangeable past incident lodged in memory. We are not. Everything I have said about strengthening the nervous system and stabilizing the mind holds good. In addition there is the old nostrum "time heals." It does, but only if we allow it to. In Western psychology one recites and reflects repeatedly on one's problems. This rumination reinforces and exacerbates the problem. While revelation can help one to see the samskara, rumination only continues to reinforce it. We all know that a scab that we constantly pick will not heal. In the same way we have to let old wounds in memory heal over. This does not mean repressing them. It means that what is not fed will wither. A sandbank that we do not add to will gradually erode. The right practice of yoga speeds this process, by enabling one to identify the impulses rising from the old imprint and by severing the mechanism that feeds it. Acting on subliminal impulses reinforces them and so the ability to intercept the rising wave is itself a progressive means of relief. As the rising impulse is stopped before causing a disturbance in our consciousness, we stop it from making a ripple on the surface that will in addition return to reinforce the sandbank at the bottom.

I can offer at least a small example from my own life. During my early travels abroad as a young man invited to spread the knowledge of yoga, I was on occasion subjected to demeaning and, to me, shocking racial discrimination. At my small hotel in London I was asked not to eat in the restaurant as it might upset the other guests, and at the airports in America, I encountered the ugly face of institutionalized racism. Although I have strong feelings about racism and equality, those incidents in no way altered my behavior or my warmth toward the people of England or the U.S.A. The wound on my youthful self left only a healthy scar, no lingering resentment, no decision to avoid such situations again by staying away. And in time laws and attitudes in those countries have changed so that others are no longer dehumanized by such arrogance and prejudice.

This principle applies to yoga's treatment of all addictions too. What we don't feed will wither. Desires, even if only expressed at a mental level, continue to nourish negative imprints. By turning our minds inward (which automatically happens) in asana and pranayama and teaching us the art of constructive action in the present moment, yoga leads consciousness away from desires and toward the inner, undisturbable core. Here, it creates a new avenue by which reflexively to perceive, observe, and recognize the heart (*antarlaksa*). In this way, the meditative mind created by yoga is a powerful therapeutic tool for removing human ills.

Memory is not a platform from which to review the world. It is a ladder whose rungs we ascend step by step. Memory is absolutely necessary for the development of intelligence. Only when intelligence (buddhi) consults memory can it get at the information it needs to initiate the transformation it seeks. While mind reacts to memory, intelligence interrogates memory. Intelligence can conduct a thorough interrogation of memory to discern consequences and make connections that mind (manas) shies away from as they are too uncomfortable. The Bhagavad Gita says that without memory, intelligence cannot prosper and so we cannot reach our soul. It is the way we use memory that is crucial, and above all which element of consciousness conducts the interview. It must be intelligence, with its power to extract the truth, reflect, and act innovatively, overriding even the mulish, recalcitrant ego.

Memory consulted by intelligence gives completely different answers to memory consulted by mind. As we have seen, memory consulted by mind and ego will always say, "What I liked give me more of, whatever the consequences. What I didn't like give me none of, whatever the consequences." Mind and memory reinvoke past experiences of pain and pleasure and equate them to the present situation, however inappropriate. Whereas intelligence makes creative comparisons, mind makes destructive ones, destructive in the sense that they fix us in a rut, an imprisoning pattern.

Memory is useful if it helps to prepare you for the future, to know whether or not you are moving forward. Use it to develop. Memory is useless if it brings about a repetition of the past. Repetition means to live in memory. If repetition is taking place, then memory retards the path of evolution. Do not live in memory. Memory is only the means to know whether we are fully aware and evolving. Never think of yesterday. Only go back if you feel that you are doing something wrong. Use yesterday's experience as a springboard. Living in the past or longing to repeat previous experience will only stagnate intelligence.

But what of the memory of the body? Does that also, like its conscious counterpart in mind have the capacity to enslave us or set us free? It does, and here again the awakening of intelligence is critical. Consciousness is potentially in every cell of our body, but most of us are comatose. The nervous system reaches everywhere. Where nerves are, mind must be. Where mind is, so is memory. Any repetitive skillful action depends on that memory. The potter's memory is in his hands. When we drive a familiar, winding road, we know instinctively how to take the bends. We do not think consciously at all. In a new stranger's house, we can never find the light switches. In our own, our hand goes to them automatically. Scents and tastes recall scenes of childhood to us without the intervention of mind.

The cellular memory also provokes negatives. "I don't want to do that. It's too much trouble." "I don't like him. He looks like my boss." Again, it is practice that brings the light of intelligence to our cells and roots out negativity. I said in chapter 2 that stretching brings the conduits of the nervous system from the center to the periphery, strengthening and relaxing them. Through these conduits (*nadi*) there is a spread of awareness. Awareness is consciousness. Intelligence is a part of consciousness and so its light is reaching every cell in areas that previously were dull and unknown to us. We hear a lot about illumination of the Soul. This is illumination of the body. Our cells die by the million every minute, but at least if we bring life to them, they live before they die. When intelligence shines into the cells, then instinct is joined by the higher faculty of intuition. Instinct is memory and mind functioning for good or ill with reference only to the past, life preserving and life destroying jumbled together. When intelligence is awakened in the cells, then instinct is transformed into intuition and the past loses its deterministic grip on us, as our inner intelligence tells us what the future requires.

Memory at the cellular level is at the service of intelligence in the form of intuition. At the conscious level it serves initially as a reference library for intelligence, to be consulted judiciously and with scholarly detachment. When intelligence consults spontaneously with memory at each moment, then conscious intuition arises, and the word we give to conscious intuition is wisdom.

There is another subtle way in which memory influences our lives without our realizing it. The imprints of memory at an unconscious level act as a filter to perception. Intelligence strives to see things as they are, but mind and memory tend to interpret these in relation to the past. The effect of this is imperceptibly to construct sandbanks of prejudice. We are all aware how prejudice acts retrospectively; you see something and place a distorted value judgment on it. But prejudice also projects itself into the future, by which I mean that it influences us to see and therefore to experience only those things that will confirm what we already think. That is why I say it acts as a filter, eliminating anything that will challenge our entrenched beliefs. If you think that all foreigners are untrustworthy, then it is certain you will meet lots of

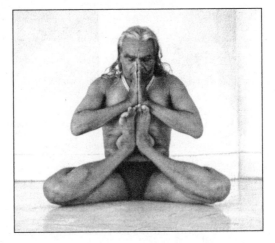

Kandasana

Chapter 5

WISDOM
The Intellectual Body (*Vijnana*)

This chapter deals with the fourth layer of our being, the Intellectual Body (*vijnanamaya kosa*), whose porous outer frontier lies next to and mingles with the Mental Body. While the mind leads to thoughts, the intellect leads to intelligence and ultimately wisdom. Yoga identifies these different parts of our consciousness, along with their accompanying fluctuations (*vrttis*) in such a way that we can use them both to give our journey direction and to result in our transformation. In this way, we discover the ability to refuse ice cream or to accept it, but in quantities that will not be harmful. We increasingly develop judicious discrimination that, harnessed to self-control, enables us to set sail in uncharted waters.

On the inner frontier of this fourth sheath lies the discovery of the individual soul (*jivatman*), that spark of divinity that resides in all of us in our Divine Body. In between these two borders of deepening self-knowledge and the culture of our higher intelligence, pure insight rests. Here comes the culmination of the exploration of the whole of our being as an individual.

This can only be accomplished by eliminating the impurities of intelligence and increasing subjugation of the cunning super ego that remains always the insecure ego, or I-Shape. The yogic tools that will facilitate this leg of our journey are the sixth and seventh petals of yoga, concentration (*dharana*) and meditation (*dhyana*). All the other petals we have studied so far, from asana to *pratyahara*, will also always be present, supporting the high achievements that to a great extent depend on them. For example, if you want to meditate, you have to sit in an asana. If you want to meditate, you have to be able to detach the mind and senses from the outer world and direct their energies inward—pratyahara. If you neglect the base, you are like someone sitting in a great tree, sawing off the branch he is sitting on.

The contents of this chapter are undoubtedly subtler, but not complicated. In fact, it is often more difficult to describe asana and *pranayama* in words than such concepts as insight, ego, and duality. The problem is rather that conscious awareness of these matters tends to lie outside our day to day experience, so they may appear abstract. They are not. They are very real. Nevertheless, an effort of imaginative intelligence is necessary to track them down and confront them.

Let me offer an analogy. Air is the element that corresponds to the sheath of intelligence, and touch is the subtle counterpart to air in our system of evolutionary theory. Imaginatively, let us explore why and how this makes sense. We bathe in air, all day and all night. Air is always against our skin. With every breath, air permeates the interior of our bodies, just as water does to a fish. Air always touches us, inwardly as well as outwardly. Touch is not only delicate, but intimate also. Do we not say about a moving experience, a book, a symphony, a film, or a meeting with someone special, "It touched me"? Air and touch go deep. And just as air surrounds and penetrates every aspect of our being and our life, so does and must intelligence. Let us see how it does so.

Examining Intelligence

We have our own individual intelligence (*buddhi*). This is the self-reflexive awareness, capable of making meaningful and freedom-enhancing choices that we met in the past chapter. It is not to be confused with *vidya* or knowledge that is acquired from external sources and remains undecided, whereas the intelligence based on our own subjective experience is an internal one and always decisive.

In this chapter, we must begin to understand that our individual intelligence, though an essential rudder to guide us, is merely a puny offshoot of cosmic intelligence (*mahat*), which is the organizing system of the universe. This intelligence is everywhere, and, like air, we constantly bathe in it and imbibe it. Of course we put barriers up against it, because we are so proud of our own individual and necessary intelligence. Thus we deprive ourselves of the full benefit of this infinite, universal, nourishing resource, just as we deprive ourselves of *pranic* energy from poor breathing. We saw how breath and consciousness go hand in hand. Similarly, individual intelligence and cosmic intelligence go hand in hand. Intelligence is the operating system of cosmic awareness.

When we eat a head of lettuce, every leaf expresses the beauty and complexity of the cosmic intelligence that formed it, and so we are partaking of cosmic intelligence by ingesting it directly. The same for each perfect grain of rice, each generous fruit. At the biological level, we are preying on them, but at the level of intelligence and consciousness, we are collaborating with them in a sacred rite, for the intelligence that organized their form and function also organized ours.

So this chapter is about moving beyond separation. It is about extension of intelligence and expansion of consciousness so that the barrier around "my" intelligence and "my" consciousness begins to dissolve. This brings the beginning of the end of loneliness. It is a fusion—or rather a transfusion—for we are transfused with the riches of natural cosmic resources. Where our common intelligence can be called "instinctive," we call this higher intelligence "insight or intuition." It penetrates barriers. The prison of particularity will soon no longer be able to hold us captive. The growth of universality will crumble its walls. As we shall see, it is meditation that crowns this process, when duality gives way to oneness. No more subject and object, this and that, me and it. It is at this point that the totality of one's being is experienced, from every cell onward, all incorporated in unique oneness, which is why it brings the vision of the individual soul. All that makes me up is now known, and I live in the awareness of the sum of its parts.

THE YOGI SAYS, according to Patanjali, in only his third *sutra*, "What reality would we see if the mind of man could still its restless waves for just an instant?" Would we be unconscious or would we be super-conscious? The answer to that is unknowable except by personal experience, which is why you can prepare for meditation, but ultimately you cannot teach it. You can do everything up to it, but it happens when it happens. You can force a piano up three flights of stairs, but you cannot force the febrile human mind to be still. All you can do is train it to be vigilant toward all that disturbs its equilibrium. That is why yoga spends so much time and effort identifying the negative, the unwanted, and the subversive, because they disturb the tranquil equilibrium of the mind. We must now explore the nature of consciousness from the viewpoint of intelligence.

The Lens of Consciousness

The meaning of *Hatha Yoga* is Sun (*Ha*) and Moon (*Tha*), Yoga in which Sun is the Soul and Moon is Consciousness. Consciousness can be compared to a lens. Its inner surface faces the soul itself, and its outer surface comes into contact with the world. Inevitably a degree of grime attaches itself to that outer surface and obscures our vision. In fact it prevents us from seeing clearly what is outside, and it equally prevents the light of our soul from shining out. If our house is gloomy because the windows are dirty, we don't say there is a problem with the sun; we clean the windows. Therefore yoga cleans the lens of consciousness in order to admit the sun (soul). So purity is not an end in itself. Similarly when a woman in India washes and says prayers before preparing food, she is purifying herself, not for the sake of purity, but to ensure that her intentions are clearly transmitted, not perverted or obscured. The loving intention behind cooking is to sustain, nourish, and uphold others. This intention can be transmitted best through a pure or clean consciousness. Clean body, clean mind, clean hands, and clean pots and pans equal a happy, healthy, loving family.

What mind is and does dies with us. But consciousness is that aspect of mind, the envelope of continual awareness, which endures, even as we believe from life to life, carrying the imprint of the past and the potential, for good or ill, of the future. Memory for past—imagination for future. Squashed between the two, we lose the ability to use direct perception on what really *is*—i.e. now, the present.

This brings us to the need to examine the nature of consciousness from a different perspective, not that of the polluting interference of the afflictions (*klesa*) that we will look at in the next chapter, but from that of five natural states or modifications of consciousness that we all experience but tend to take for granted. Yoga says there is much to be learned from them as they too are patterns of thought waves that influence the mind and its ability to perceive truly. If the reader is puzzled by this insistence on examining the myriad waves of thought that ruffle the lake of consciousness, let me just remind you again of Patanjali's second *sutra*, "Yoga is the stilling of the fluctuations of consciousness." Why? Because yoga is meditation, and this chapter is about concentration and meditation. A ruffled mind cannot meditate, which is why we must identify and pacify all disturbing patterns. The consciousness must become passively alert—not placid like a cow contentedly chewing the cud, but alert and receptive like a wild deer in the forest, except that whereas the deer's senses are turned outward, the yogi's, with equal acuity, are directed inward. This is intelligence enthroned in awareness, about to enter the mystery of the unknown. Yet our consciousness is not always alert, and so we must explore the modifications of our mind that prevent us from having this acuity.

Transforming the Mind

Consciousness (*citta*) has three functions. The first is *cognition*, which is perceiving, knowing, and recognizing. The second is *volition*, or will, which is the impulse to initiate action. The third is *motion*, which expresses the fire nature of mind, ever transforming itself and leaping up in different places and guises. These all serve for us to gain knowledge and appreciate the truth concerning humankind's position in the universe.

Let us look at the fiery nature of mind. Fire flickers and dances, so does mind. In fact, consciousness modifies itself so rapidly that before we can recognize one fluctuation and examine it, it gets muddled with another. These muddled changes are a natural process. They show the vivacity of consciousness. All our activities depend upon these mental fluctuations.

I have said that mind dances. It would also be true to say that mind leads us on a merry dance. If you want to get the best out of a fiery horse, you have to understand, tame, and control it. The same is true for a fiery mind, or it will run away with you. Because mind is always drawn outward by the senses into the attractions of the material world, it cannot help but land us into a lot of tricky situations, ones we had not bargained for, or that look good at first but turn sour on us.

The way Patanjali expressed this is to say that the fluctuations of consciousness can be either painful or nonpainful, either visible or invisible. He meant that some things look unpleasing, distressing, anguishing, and they are. Studying for an exam can be very hard. The benefits of passing the exam remain hidden, invisible until later. Conversely, the joys of the table are extremely pleasant, and the pains and problems that result from overindulgence may remain invisible for a long time. If eventually an illness or debility results, then that is a visible pain. But if we use all our resources, courage, will, and faith to overcome the sickness, a nonpainful state emerges again. This is a way of warning us that there are always two sides to every coin and that we should be guarded and thoughtful before we rush into things. There is always a price to pay or a reward to be earned. But the phrase "If it feels good, do it" is not a maxim to be trusted in the long run. All philosophies recognize that a pleasure-seeker will end up as a pain-finder. The ancient Greeks said that moderation was the greatest virtue. Yoga says that it is through practice and detachment that we learn to avoid ricocheting from one extreme of pleasure and pain to the other.

This double aspect of the fluctuating mind applies to what are called the Five Modifications of Consciousness (in Sanskrit called *citta vrittis*). These are correct knowledge (*pramana*), wrong knowledge or misconception (*viparyaya*), imagination or fantasy (*vikalpa*), sleep (*nidra*), and memory (*smrti*). These are natural psychological states that occur in everyone. They are dependent on the brain and nervous system and disappear at death. One might be forgiven for wondering what the point is of studying them. Sleep is sleep, imagination is imagination, and as regards the first two, well, sometimes I'm right, and sometimes I'm wrong. Yet from the yogic standpoint, there is a huge value in understanding them. Their misuse when they are defective can lead to endless trouble. They affect both the quality of our life and the actions we perform in it. The consequences of our actions endure. The implications are karmic. "As you sow, so shall you reap." This is a universal understanding. Yoga does not limit consequences to this life only. How does someone who is wrong about everything, lives in fantasies, sleeps badly, and misuses memory conduct himself? Hitler truly believed that the Jewish people were subhuman and acted accordingly. This was wrong knowledge or misperception, total delusion. The consequence in his lifetime was his death and his country's destruction along with much of the world. If the chain of causality does survive the grave, would anyone like to exchange places with Hitler now?

It is definitely worth looking at these five forms of consciousness in both their beneficial and deficient aspects. Their study can help us to follow a certain way of life and adopt a right way of thinking. They show us a direction and enable us to channel the thinking process. Our aim is not to arrest or restrain them but gradually to transform them. They are not separate but intertwined like threads in a cloth. One affects the others. The dullness of poor quality or *tamasic* sleep degrades the clarity of the four other modifications. Sharp analysis for right knowledge becomes impossible. When you are tired, it is not easy to remember things. We also depend on memory to recall all other states. It links and underpins them.

In the past chapter, we looked at the two aspects of memory, one damaging, the other liberating. We saw that the "painful" form of memory brings bondage in psychological time, condemning us to relive the past in endless, meaningless permutations. We are like a cart in the monsoon, its wheels bogged down in mud. The "painless" form is discrimination (*viveka*), essential for our growth.

Discrimination is the knife edge of intellect, separating true from false, reality from unreality, using memory in such a way that past consequences are factored into our choices and decisions. If we can see consequences, we are not caught in the trap of apparent pain versus apparent pleasure. Discrimination is about making meaningful comparisons such as, "How does my practice compare with that of yesterday?" or "How does the stretch on my left leg compare with that on my right?" You may well find the right leg is asleep. Initially, this is a process of trial and error. Later we can learn to avoid error. In headstand pose, for example, something that usually goes wrong is that the upper arm shortens. Memory warns us to be careful before that happens. In this way, we break down bad habits. This is a useful discrimination that awakens awareness.

Awareness, working with discrimination and memory, encourages a creative mind, not a mechanical one. The mechanical mind questions only external phenomena, treating the world like a giant machine and resulting in objective knowledge. By objective knowledge I mean knowledge of the world around us. This can be useful or dangerous, depending on how you use it. Comparing your neighbor's new car to your old one may lead to jealousy and covetousness, or it might lead you to appreciate that his is safer or causes less pollution. But what I call the creative brain calls into question both the outer and inner, leading us to subjective and spiritual knowledge. By subjective knowledge I mean knowledge of oneself from the skin inward. To take the example of your neighbor's car, if you have understood that pollution is undesirable, you will not want to pollute the atmosphere (outer) or pollute yourself (inner). So a creative reaction might be to change your car.

When awareness is linked to intelligence, we are able to see with absolute honesty. When brain and body move in harmony, there is integrity. Memory supports this process because when memory functions perfectly, it becomes one with intelligence. By transferring its allegiance from the pleasure-seeking mind to the discerning intelligence, memory no longer digs pits of old habit for us to fall into but becomes our true guru by guiding us toward perfect knowledge and behavior.

By purifying memory, we purify our whole mind. For an average person, memory is a past state of mind. For the yogi, it is a present state of mind. We should not forget that memory records everything. Memory is useless if it brings about a repetition of the past that impedes the process of our evolution. But memory is useful if it helps to prepare you for the future and even necessary if you use it to develop. Memory is a continuous profit and loss account through which we can see whether we are receding or proceeding. By sorting out wanted from unwanted memory, we allow new experiences to surface. The whole of the useful past is now at our present disposition. Memory ceases to function as a separate entity and merges with consciousness. Patanjali said that when memory is cleansed completely, the mind drops like the ripe fruit and consciousness shines in its purest form. By this I mean that when memory serves as a spur to perfect present action without taint, then it is acting in its intended form. A cleansed memory is one that does not contain undigested emotions from the unconscious but that deals with feelings in the present as they arise.

Imagination too can work either to our benefit or to our detriment. It is undoubtedly the greatest gift to human beings. But the Sanskrit word vikalpa also means fantasy or delusion. Without steady application, even the most inspiring flights of imagination must remain impotent, devoid of reality. If a scientist has an idea, he may have to labor for years, experimenting, analyzing, and checking in order to bring it to fruition, to make it concrete. A writer may dream of the plot for a new novel, but unless he applies himself to pen and paper, his ideas have no value. A callow youth once said to a great poet, "I have a marvelous idea for a new poem." The poet replied cuttingly, "Poems are about words." The true poet had his feet on the ground. Never mind the idea, write it down.

You can see how the five modifications combine against us. When we daydream, we are mixing fantasy and the dullness of sleep. If we are daydreaming about the past, we add memory to the mixture. This may be pleasant and soothing, but it leads nowhere. In fact, when we return to present reality, we may find it, by comparison, quite unpalatable. This is a painful state emerging from a painless one.

Those who fail to emerge from solely imaginative thoughts never command respect; they remain lightweights. We reserve our greatest respect for those who transform a panoramic and penetrating vision into reality. As a young man, Mahatma Gandhi imagined an India independent and free of British rule, yet it took him a lifetime of unremitting labor, of *tapas*, to realize his dream. Tapas is the key here. The word implies intense, purifying heat, a fire that, like the alchemist's, transforms base metal into gold. Imagination is the flickering flame, the coolest part of the fire. Dancing flames give light to reveal shape, which in yoga terminology is the subtle counterpart of fire. What is an idea, a concept, but a shape in the mind? The work before us is to blow on the fire with the bellows of tapas, so that it becomes intensely hot and transforms the shapes of mind into reality. Asana practice brings mind and body into harmony for this task. Your mind is always ahead of your body. The mind moves into the future, the body the past, but the self is in the present. The coordination between them that we learn in asana will enable us to turn the shape of our visions into the substance of our lives.

Sleep is sleep. I asked earlier, "What can it teach us?" After all, we never witness it. We are inert and unconscious and have no direct memory of it. Yet we always know how we have slept. Deep dreamless, nourishing sleep is worth hoping for. Yogis do not dream. Either they are in sleep or awake. Sleep is of three types. If one feels heavy and dull after sleep, then that sleep has been tamasic. Disturbed, agitated sleep is *rajasic*. Sleep that brings lightness, brightness, and freshness is *sattvic*. Sleep, to use the metaphor again, is like an open rose returning to the bud. The senses of perception rest in the mind, the mind in the consciousness, the consciousness in the being. This sounds like a description of exactly what we are trying to achieve through yoga, so surely there is something to be learned. We even return to innocence in sleep. No sleeper can be a sinner.

Because the mind and senses are at rest, a negative state of void exists, a feeling of emptiness or absence. It can be described as negative because the present and aware state of consciousness is absent. The goal of the student of yoga is to transform this into a positive state of mind while awake. The senses and the mind close up like a bud, but a witness remains alert. This is a pure state in which the self is free from the accumulations of experience. The movements of consciousness are calmed. Peaceful deep sleep, experienced while alert and awake, is *samadhi*. When the mind is controlled and still, what remains is the soul. The absence of ego in the state of sleep is akin to samadhi, but it is dull and without awareness. Samadhi is the egolessness of sleep combined with the vibrancy of intelligence.

When we are in deep sleep, we lose our ego, our "I-ness." We forget who we are and return to the cosmic, eternal mind. There is a brief moment on awaking, before "I"-consciousness returns, when we can just glimpse this tranquil, egoless state. It should be our guide. It is a natural window onto the meditative mind in which we realize that we are one and learn to accept. When the ego is quiescent, our sense of pride lessens. We are receptive and become more understanding. We are not offended by life's affronts. We become insulated from anxiety and anguish both within and without.

The practice of yoga teaches us to deal with each task in the day as it arises, and then to put it down. This might include answering our letters or returning our calls, doing the washing up, letting anger drop as soon as the moment is past. There is an old phrase "Sufficient to the day the evils thereof." It means we should contain even disagreeable challenges of life in their appropriate place and not let them fester and pollute the rest of our time. If we learn this, our sleep will not carry over a toxic hangover from the previous day of unresolved worries and fears. Similarly, we should not eat heavily or too late as our sleep will be turbulent (rajasic). We will awake in a discontented, agitated state. If we feed our minds on violent images, thoughts, and words, our unconscious will regurgitate them in disturbed dreams. Just as right imagination opens the creative mind, right sleep exhilarates the mind and brings alertness. By living each day presently and thoroughly, we earn a clear conscience. A clear conscience is the best preparation for a restful and peaceful night.

It is sometimes said that a dullard, someone who is completely vacuous, presents to the observer the same appearance as one who is in samadhi, a state of divine bliss. This is because neither the dullard's mind, nor the saint's, has movement in the consciousness. The difference is that one is negative, comatose, and insensitive, but the other is alert, positive, and supremely aware. I mention this because it is easy for beginners to confuse somnolence or a pleasant languor with the meditative state. Often, as students do *Savasana* (corpse pose, see chapter 7) or attempt meditation, they drift into an agreeable torpor, as if they were swaddled in cotton wool. This is not the prelude to samadhi but to sleep. The dullness of sleep is undesirable in a waking state. So is the frenetic overactivity that arises from turbulent sleep. If we toss and turn at night, we shall toss and turn in the day. What we are seeking is an alert, self-contained, egoless state that corresponds to the refreshing aftermath of good repose. The experience of repose at night will give us clues to the repose of mind and sense in the meditative state. Good sleep makes consciousness brilliant. Poor sleep leaves it tarnished.

A bad night makes us see everything askew. Erroneous knowledge gives rise to erroneous thought, words, and action. They are not harmless. Often, when we correct our misperceptions, we look back and say, "I shouldn't have said that," or "I shouldn't have done this." We feel guilt and regret. Yet in the practical world, we put a lot of effort into avoiding this situation. If we are buying a house, we employ a surveyor to check its structure, the safety of the land, and the supply of water, and we hire a title company to verify the legal deeds, and we ask a bank to carry out the financial transaction correctly. We check availability of schools and transport. We don't want to make a mistake. Yet most people, looking back on their lives, see them as being littered with mistakes.

We say, "If only I'd known then what I know now." But what we know now does not seem to stop us from making more mistakes. The yogic blueprint says that right knowledge and erroneous knowledge are two modifications, or states, of consciousness. By the practice of yoga, we can lessen and eradicate misperception and wrong knowledge and gain accurate perception and right knowledge. I am not talking about changing our opinions, although this may happen, but rather about abandoning them altogether. An opinion is yesterday's right or wrong knowledge warmed up and re-served for today's situation. So opinions are rooted in the past, and our examination of memory has shown us that the past can be a minefield. The practitioner of yoga is always trying to be in the present, which is where reality is, and so perfect present awareness in a given situation is his goal. This is not to be reached in one bound. So one of the things we may notice about ourselves on the Inward Journey is that opinions based on wrong perception and information are gradually replaced by those with a more accurate foundation. This is akin to a situation when we changed bad habits into good ones prior to reaching an unconditioned freedom. Let us look at an example.

Thirty or forty years ago, most people held the view that women were not able to do men's jobs, that they were more suited to subservient tasks, and that even if they did a man's job, they should receive less pay. Most people no longer believe this. The climate of opinion has changed. And we would say that the current evidence confirms our change of opinion. We consider this progress away from erroneous knowledge. It is based on actual evidence of how women perform in the workplace and so is less shackled to prejudice. Prejudice means making up your mind before you look.

During this process of change, if a man and a woman came to you for a job, you might have been inclined, all other things being equal, to favor the woman, consciously trying to act out of the new view of women's capabilities and perhaps to redress past injustice. But if you favor the woman when the candidates are equal, you are still acting out of prejudice. The past still has its hold. You have effectively turned a bad habit into a "better" one, but where is the right action, based on right knowledge, without previous conditioning? In this example, presumably the solution is to be able to interview the candidates with such clarity of vision as regards their abilities and suitability, that a choice emerges, but without any shadow of reference to their gender.

This example is external. Yogic practice is internal. What we have to look at is how the culture of the self leads to direct, right knowledge that then inevitably reforms and transforms our relationship with the external world as well as furthering our inner quest.

ACCORDING TO YOGA PHILOSOPHY, correct knowledge is based on three kinds of proof: direct perception, correct deduction, and testimony from authoritative sacred scriptures or wise experienced people. Initially, therefore, individual perception should be checked by logic and reason and then seen to correspond to traditional wisdom. We are all familiar with this process. In the example of buying a house, we see the house and form an impression (our direct perception). We then make an assessment based on what we learn about the house (hopefully correct deduction). The surveyor is our experienced sage, and his technical reference books are the scriptures. In this way, the three kinds of proof ideally corroborate one another.

The faculty you are using here is intelligence (buddhi), which we saw in the past chapter to be more subtle than the thinking, sensorial brain (*manas*). It is concerned with facts and reason, not impressions and interpretations. It is inherent in every aspect of our being but tends to remain dormant, so our first step is to tap it and awaken it.

The practice of asana brings intelligence to the surface of the cellular body through stretching and to the physiological body through maintaining the asana. Once awakened, the body can reveal its dynamic aspect, its ability to discriminate. Here the body is providing subjective factual truth while the mind is generating imaginative ideas. It is the precise, thorough measuring and adjustment of a pose, bringing balance, stability, and equal extension everywhere that hones this faculty of discrimination. Discrimination is a weighing process, belonging to the world of duality. When what is wrong is discarded, what is left must be correct. As intelligence expands in consciousness, then ego and mind contract to their proper proportions. They no longer rule the roost, but serve intelligence. Memory, especially, as we have seen, is now harnessed to the freedom-seeking intelligence, not the bondage-seeking mind.

Prajna—Insight and Intuition

There is a further stage. Spiritual intelligence, which is true wisdom, dawns only when discrimination ends. Wisdom does not function in duality. It perceives only oneness. It does not discard the wrong; it sees and feels only the right. When we are buying a house, we need to use the logical, discriminating intelligence. A politician, however high his motives, must choose and decide in the relative and temporal world. Spiritual wisdom, on the other hand, does not decide, it knows. It is entirely present and so is free of time, as we shall see as we move inward closer to the soul.

For the moment we must be content to see the sky clearly and say that it is blue when the sun shines. Ultimately, science tells us, the atmosphere is colorless, like water. Sensory perception may be flawed, but at least clear, healthy senses will show us the wonderful variety of color in the sky or in the waters of rivers and lakes. This knowledge is not perfect, but it is valid. It provides a reasonable foundation. A good nervous system will make our actions swift and sure. Healthy bodies give strength to act; unclouded minds give stability and relief from emotional upheavals. The awakening of intelligence will help us to choose, decide, and initiate action. What we are witnessing is a coming together, an integration, of the sheaths of being that we are exploring, so that they can act in harmony and from a source that is moving ever closer to the core.

What I am describing here is a journey from a chattering brain to clean instinct to reach the clarity of intuition. When you start yoga, you probably are living in your mind and emotions, a never-ending Internet chat room. You read books and articles on what best to eat and how to exercise, reading material that any wild animal would scorn. But you do not know how to live, only what you desire. Instinct is dulled. With asana and pranayama practice, first we move outward from mind and cleanse the body, senses, and organs. Instinct is revitalized. The newly awoken intelligence of the body moves in and tells you automatically what food is good for you, when and how much to eat, when and how to exercise, and when to rest or sleep. People forget that in our quest for the soul, we first reclaim the pristine joys of the animal kingdom, health and instinct, vibrant and alive. At the same time, we are transforming instinct into intuition. Intelligence cuts its teeth on analysis and synthesis, reason and deduction. It becomes muscular. And gradually the higher intelligence of intuition begins to dawn, like light in the sky before sunrise. Instinct is the unconscious intelligence of the cells surfacing. Intuition is supra-conscious knowing in which you know before you know *how* you know.

When I was young, I used to travel by train from Pune to Bombay every weekend to teach. The train I took was the race special for the horse race meeting in Bombay. Crowded together, all the race goers assumed I was off to the races too. I got tired of explaining otherwise and often passengers would ask me what I thought of a particular race, offering me the list of runners. Quickly I would name a horse. It was astonishing how many returning punters would approach me and say, "You know, that horse you picked won!" It was probably chance, but I give the example lightheartedly to show that this is how intuition dawns. Little things turn out to be spontaneously correct. We find ourselves putting round pegs into round holes, and square pegs in square ones. We are mentally less clumsy, more adroit.

Sustained misperception and wrong knowledge lead to a life of trying to hammer square pegs into round holes, or in racing terms, picking losers. If you persist in hammering, it can lead to disastrous results, for you and for others. Confusion, mixing things up, and mistaking one for another is the opposite of discrimination. Misconception creates a distortion of reality that in turn generates wrong feelings and taints the consciousness. By culturing intelligence and learning from mistakes, we weed out what is wrong. Any gardener will tell you that weeds grow back, but at least they are easier to dig up if we catch them before they are fully grown.

We have now discussed how to develop our individual intelligence in our lives. As we move farther inward through the intellectual sheath, this intelligence is cultivated into wisdom. Here we will see the importance that concentration and meditation play in culturing the mind. By moving ever away from the understandable but often childish promptings of ego, we turn our source of knowing from our brains to our hearts and from our minds to our souls. Just as our souls are part of a Universal Soul, we have also seen that our intelligence is part of a Universal Intelligence. As we learn to attune ourselves like an antenna to this natural intelligence around us, we gain not just clarity of thought but also wisdom in life. We are able to develop ever greater access to this wisdom as we learn to develop right perception. We are also much more likely to perceive this wisdom as we learn to transform the dull, distracted, or oscillating mind into an attentive and restrained yogic mind.

The Five Qualities of Mind (*Bhumis*)

In order to make us more aware of consciousness as an ocean with wave patterns constantly moving across it, yoga has highlighted five calibers or qualities of mind that correspond to the five modifications we have been discussing. They include a dull state, a distracted monkey mind, an alternating or oscillating mind, a single-pointed attentive mind, and finally the highest stage, the restrained consciousness that is experienced in the timeless state of absorption we call samadhi.

These calibers of consciousness are aids to self-observation and self-knowledge, not accusations of mental debility. There is a popular misconception that yoga is only for those who have power of concentration. But all of us are not so endowed. Yoga can be practiced by anyone, whatever one's state of mind or health. It is through practice that the scattered mind is brought to a focal point (knee, chest, etc.). This is a training regimen that moves us toward direct perception. Humor helps people move from fragmentation to wholeness too. It lightens the mind and makes it easier to guide and focus. A stable mind is like the hub of a wheel. The world may spin around you, but the mind is steady.

Humorists are very observant of fluctuating consciousness. Their subject matter is frequently dull or silly people, or those with wandering minds, constantly making illogical jumps and associations. Humorists cleverly show how ridiculous this is. And all the time the humorist is mimicking the dull and distracted, he himself is acutely concentrated on presenting his material. And as we laugh and lighten our minds, we in turn concentrate on every word he is saying. Clever people make fortunes out of understanding the tricks of mind. Artists too are aware of the caliber of consciousness of their audience. An English writer said two hundred years ago that there are four classes of reader. The first he compares to an hourglass; their reading being as the sand; it runs in and runs out and leaves not a vestige behind. A second class resembles a sponge, which imbibes everything and returns it in nearly the same state, only a little dirtier. A third class he likens to a jelly bag, which allows all that is pure to pass away and retains all the refuse and the dregs. The fourth class may be compared to the slaves in the diamond mines of Golconda, who, casting aside all that is worthless, preserve only the pure gems.

As it happens, the diamond mines of Golconda are not very far from where I was born. But what, in yogic terms and at this fourth level of our being that we are examining, do we mean by diamonds? Diamonds are hard and clear. It is their property of clarity that gives us the clue. Clarity is also the great defining characteristic of wisdom. We are seeking to cultivate wisdom, to transform mental dexterity or cleverness, which all people possess in some degree, into the penetrating clear light of wisdom.

In order to achieve this, we have to toil in the mines, to separate dross, which is false, from what is precious because it is true. Let us look at this sifting process through the example of yoga practice.

The Culture of Intelligence

I sometimes tell my pupils that the practice they do in yoga class is not, strictly speaking, yoga practice. The reason for this is that in a class, although you are undoubtedly "doing" and, hopefully, learning you are subordinate to the teacher. The directing intelligence comes from him, and you follow to the best of your ability. At home, on the other hand, it is your own intelligence that is the master, and the progress that you make is yours and will be maintained. In addition, the will that you employ is yours. It is not derived from the power, the charisma, the strength, or the fieriness of the teacher. It comes from you, and its effect profound. This is not yoga *by* the body *for* the body, but yoga *by* the body *for* the mind, *for* the intelligence.

There is a great difference between just practicing and *sadhana*. Sadhana is the way of accomplishing something. That something is— by effective performance and correct execution—the achievement of the real. What is real must be true and so lead us toward purity and emancipation. This is *yoga sadhana* and not the mechanical repetition merely of yoga practice or *yogabhyasa*. The end of yoga sadhana is wisdom. You might translate yoga sadhana here as "the yoga pilgrimage" as it is a journey that leads somewhere, not the mere treadmill of thoughtless practice.

When I say a phrase like "wisdom comes from culturing the intelligence," everybody nods in agreement, but really we are in danger of overinflating our minds. So let us just pause to steady ourselves, as we do in asana, and explore what we mean by intelligence.

For example, one root way to grasp its meaning is to say that intelligence is sensitivity in the body that is felt by the consciousness and conscience. Conscience is very close to the Self, as we will see shortly. Through the sensitivity you gain in asana practice, you can also diagnose where sensation is absent. This is the function of intelligence, sifting the earth in the mines of Golconda. Its next function is to bring sensation to where it is not, and to make awareness flow there too. And when sensation is general, you are a sensate being, which means that you are alive—perhaps for the first time since your birth. Beyond that, you have to observe whether the sensitivity is equally distributed or not. Intelligence here is the will to alter where it finds imperfections. The rapid, dexterous mind works in the service of intelligence, training itself to collect its scattered thoughts and apply itself to the greater good, which is the good of the Whole. Mind is necessary to fabricate the grammar, syntax, and vocabulary with which we establish relations with other forms of life. Even the highest form of intelligence should not forget to be grateful to its feeling, gathering mind, for it needs, above all, to borrow the words and grammar afforded by mind in order to express itself outwardly.

At this level of practice, where total attention is almost within our grasp and total penetration is becoming a real possibility, there is something of a parting of the ways concerning what is called Free Will. Free Will for most people implies being able, for good or ill, to do what we want and not do what we don't. Our yoga practice up till now will have enhanced these potentials. Growing health, vigor, brightness, and self-control will have enabled us to take on more and different activities than before, change the quality of our relationships, and of course, put the ice cream back in the freezer. All this comes into most people's idea of self-realization, and it is a pleasant and essential aspect of living one's life. But now another side to Free Will is beginning to declare itself, and you might call that "The Will to be Free." In spite of its attractive sound, it is, to the average person, a daunting prospect, implying as it does, penetration into the heart of the unknown, detachment, and the potential pain of ultimate self-knowledge. This requires real guts, and so we should take a moment to look at the source of our will.

In 1944, I struggled terribly with my practice. It was dry, lifeless, and artificial. I was acting from the will of my head, my ego, and not from my heart, my intelligence. The simple fact is that the will of the ego is finite, because our ego is finite. It is a personal attribute, limited to us. It is just the sum of all our past experiences and acquisitions. Coming from the head, it will always feel forced. Coming from a finite origin, it will always eventually run out.

The will that springs from the intelligence of the heart is, by contrast, linked to an infinite resource—cosmic intelligence (mahat) and cosmic consciousness. It is a well that will never run dry. Yoga calls the will, or incitement to action, that derives from universal consciousness *prerana*. People who are addicted to drugs or alcohol are encouraged not to do what is called "white knuckle self-control," as its egoic source will eventually be exhausted and a crash will follow. On the contrary, they are told to "hand over to a higher power," which means that their will is replenished every day through contact with the cosmic source of intelligent action. Prerana, which I touched on in chapter 2, is the intelligent will of Nature's consciousness expressing itself through us. And it expresses itself through the heart, not the head. It is by tapping the source of infinite will and intelligence that we discover in ourselves the guts to penetrate the inner recesses of our Being.

The intelligence we are now developing depends upon emotional and moral maturity, the ability to value truth and respect ethical conduct, the capacity to feel love in its more universal sense as compassion. I referred to Socrates in the introduction in relation to the philosophical injunction to "know thyself." But what is now revealed as the value of knowing yourself? It must have some point. Socrates said quite simply that self-knowledge allows us to live *deliberately* out of a state of freedom. The analogy I offer to explain the significance of the word deliberately is that most of us travel through life in the same way an eighteen-month-old baby walks. The reason he keeps putting one foot in front of the other is that if he doesn't, he will fall over. His walk is a sustained totter, punctuated by falls. To live deliberately is to walk like an adult, to have balance, direction, and purpose and to walk in growing freedom and assurance toward the ultimate freedom.

Sanskrit etymology throws light on the point we have now reached. I have just said that we are learning to walk as adults. Well, in Sanskrit, *Maanava* means man. By association with manas, it also means one who has a mind. And another meaning of *maana* is to live with honor and dignity. The implication is clear. We are human beings, gifted with intelligence that lends purpose and direction to our steps, striving to live ethically, that is with honor and dignity.

The question that hangs over mankind is, "Can we really achieve freedom?" We often hold the contradictory notion in our heads that Gandhi or Jesus or Aurobindo reached freedom, but that we cannot. And our daily experience, our failures and disappointments, only seem to confirm our prejudice against ourselves. But read the life of Gandhi, of Aurobindo. Their lives were full of setbacks, wrong paths embarked upon, even early immorality. I have already made clear that the basis of my life in yoga was sickliness, ostracism, ridicule, and my general uselessness for any other path in life.

To resolve this paradox, we have to cast our minds back to the relationship between Nature (*Prakrti*) and Soul (*Purusa*). Here we have to discriminate between determinism and inevitability. We are biologically determined by nature for our own evolutionary benefit. At the biological level, this determinism is so strong that it creates inevitability—i.e. we all have two arms, two legs, and one head, etc. At the level of consciousness, deterministic forces produce a strong predisposition in us, for example, to repeat pleasure, avoid pain, flee what we fear, and allow ego and pride to swell. But this is *not* inevitable. It is merely an unlevel playing field. Yoga is a thoroughly tested technique whereby the Will, working through an intelligence that can choose and a self-aware consciousness, can free us from inevitability. By these means, we can walk deliberately toward an individual emancipation and, by the grace of Heaven, a universal freedom.

It is said that Adam and Eve lived in a state of primal or original Oneness. Yoga says that the highest experience of freedom is Oneness, the supreme reality of Unity. The predicament of human beings is that we feel ourselves to be stuck in a no-man's-land between the beginning and the end of an immense journey. Adam and Eve took the first step toward individuation when they ate the forbidden fruit and lost their primal unity. We are still carrying on their arduous journey. We cannot go back. Where we are is uncomfortable—so we must go on. On the way we will taste both the sweet and bitter fruits of individuation, and they will be included and integrated in our experience of the journey toward full consciousness. But nothing says we cannot reach the goal of Oneness, Paradise Regained, a final, not a primal, Unity. To make such a long journey, we need power—in fact we need three powers (*sakti*).

Power and Wisdom—*Sakti*

Now it is time to go back to our own origins in yoga practice in order to further our inward journey. We have established through practice, but must not neglect, the power of a healthy body (*sarira sakti*). But a body without energy and consciousness is half dead. In chapter 3 on pranayama, we established the vital importance of the power of pranic energy (*prana sakti*). Now I introduce another power, that of awareness (*prajna*). Prajna is awareness of consciousness. I mentioned it only a few paragraphs ago as self-aware consciousness but did not give the Sanskrit translation. The power of self-awareness is prajna sakti. Prajna is also translated as knowledge of wisdom.

These three powers have first to be brought into alignment in order to coordinate with the power of the soul (*atma sakti*) so that they may merge with it. Body power plus energy can, as I warned in chapter 3, overload the system by putting too high a voltage through an inadequate circuit. It is by adding the power of the awareness of consciousness that we balance these huge forces within us. This makes possible expansion at every level (*kosa*) but without danger, strain, or overload. The role of awareness is to fill the gaps that inevitably exist between the physical (bones, muscles, etc.) and organic (e.g. organs) sheaths of our bodies when we practice asana. Even when we are integrating the various sheaths of our bodies there are gaps that we fail to fill with awareness and energy. The constant practice of all petals of yoga will eventually repair all flaws inherent within the human system. The power we generate through yoga practice must become a coherent and indissoluble whole. Yoga sadhana is meant to knit the fibers to the skin and skin to the fibers so that they coil and interweave the outer kosa into the *atma kosa*. Only then can the Oneness of the power we create within ourselves be integrated with the universal power that surrounds us. If not, divisions will inevitably remain.

I have talked in this chapter of mahat (cosmic intelligence), existing as a universal resource at our disposition. Prajna sakti, the power of awareness, is nothing less than cosmic intelligence seeping and soaking into the dark spaces of our being to illuminate them with consciousness. Consciousness has to settle down with clarity, brightness, and serenity. This renders a gratifying satisfaction to the conscience that is egoless and very close to the Soul.

In practical terms, how does this work? We already know that cosmic energy (*prana*) is carried into us by the vehicle of breath. So how is cosmic awareness inducted into us? What fuels it? The fuel is willpower or sustained intention with attention. See how we are moving closer to concentration (dharana), the sixth petal of yoga? But still you must be asking, "How do I ignite the fuel of my willpower? I know it comes from the heart, not the head, but I cannot just conjure it up from thin air!" Yes you can—for it is air, or rather prana, which ignites the fuel of will and allows awareness to spread and percolate throughout our systems. Energy and awareness (both cosmic entities) act as friends. Where one goes, the other follows. It is by the will of awareness to penetrate that intelligence is able to move into and occupy the darkest inner recesses of our being. This intelligence is clarity to lighten the darkness. This is the dawn of wisdom, the intuitive insight that sees because it sees, knows because it knows, and acts immediately and spontaneously because the three powers of body, energy, and awareness have merged and aligned themselves with the light emitted by the soul. We say intelligence has insight. We should complement that by saying that the soul has "outsight;" it is a beacon shining out. As I said at the beginning of the book, during the Inward Journey, as our Will goes inward our Soul comes outward to meet us.

I have talked a lot on freedom, from various angles. Something we all associate with freedom is space. Americans refer nostalgically to the space and freedom of the Old West. Space is freedom, and we create, like a big bang, space within by the practice of asana and pranayama. A dark space is unknown and unknowing (*avidya*). But when the power of energy and the power of awareness combine, there is a flash of lightning that banishes darkness. It is by the exercise of our drive toward consciousness that we witness this. It is a subjective revelation as no one else can witness it, or corroborate it, but is it not also true that if you have a toothache, no one else can feel it, yet no authority on earth can convince you that your tooth does not hurt?

We use the phrase "the inward journey" a lot throughout this book. Now we find ourselves in a realm where the inner is visibly trying to get out, to express itself. The space we create is such that the source body, the innermost, can begin to radiate out. If your practice remains only at the physical level, the space essential to liberate the inner will be missing. The realization that each cell has its own intelligence through which to realize its brief existence will never come. You will remain locked in the dark density of matter, when what you are seeking is for that inner light to irradiate space. It is a shame to practice yoga so much and to this level, yet still remain encumbered with ego. One should be natural, like a happy, confident child. The soul seeks nothing more than to expand to fill our whole being. But still we maintain an internal cringe, a sense of unworthiness, which often we mask by a projection of an arrogant, false personality. This is just one of the inherent flaws that exist equally in intelligence.

Impurities of Intelligence

The whole educative thrust of yoga is to make things go right in our lives. But we all know that an apple that appears perfect on the outside can have been eaten away by an invisible worm on the inside. Yoga is not about appearances. It is about finding and eradicating the worm, so that the whole apple, from skin inward, can be perfect and a healthy one. That is why yoga, and indeed all spiritual philosophies, seems to harp on the negative—grasping desires, weaknesses, faults, and imbalances. They are trying to catch the worm before it devours and corrupts the whole apple from inside. This is not a struggle between good and evil. It is natural for worms to eat apples. In yoga we simply do not want to be the apple that is rotted from inside. So yoga insists on examining, scientifically and without value judgment, what can go wrong, and why, and how to stop it. It is organic farming of the self—for the Self.

To reach and penetrate as far as the fourth sheath is a considerable achievement, but I would be doing the reader a disservice if I did not point out that considerable achievements also bring in their wake considerable dangers. An obvious one is pride—not satisfaction in a job well done—but a sense of superiority and difference, of distinction and eminence.

It is an obsession in our modern society to focus on appearance, presentation, and packaging. We do not ask ourselves, "How am I really?" but "How do I look, how do others see me?" It is not a question of, "What am I saying?" but, "How do I sound?"

There are those, for example, who perform polished, well-presented, highly attractive *yogasana*. They are pleased with this, and with themselves, and are perhaps financially well rewarded for this outward excellence. When I was young, struggling to earn a living, to raise yoga in public esteem, to exemplify in my visible body the art and aesthetic beauty of yoga, I was always seeking to present asana in the best possible way, symmetrically, precisely, and in stimulating, coherent sequences. I was, when occasion demanded, a performer and an artist. This was my service to the art of yoga. But in my own personal practice I did not have this type of idea. I was concerned only to explore, to learn, to challenge, and to transform inwardly. Above all to penetrate. Yoga is an interior penetration leading to integration of being, senses, breath, mind, intelligence, consciousness, and Self. It is definitely an inward journey, evolution through involution, toward the Soul, which in its turn desires to emerge and embrace you in its glory.

You need a good teacher as guide so you will not hurt your body, overstretch, wrench, or nip the inner fibers, tendons, ligaments, mind, and emotions. This is yoga inadequately or wrongly practiced. I know; I have done it. But when yoga is only outward facing, exhibitative, and self-gratifying, it is not yoga at all. Such an attitude will deface and deform even the character you started out with. In class when pride rises or its complement, insecurity, as you look around at others, recognize it for what it is and send it on its way.

It is certain that there is much pleasure and satisfaction to be gleaned from life. Patanjali said the correct fulfillment of pleasure is an essential component not only of life but of liberation. But Patanjali also warned that wrong interaction with nature (where the afflictions or klesa still rule us) can bring about our confusion and self-destruction. The pursuit of pleasure through appearances, which I connect here to superficiality of intent, is quite simply the wrong way to go about things. To pursue pleasure is to pursue pain in equal measure. When appearance is more important to us than content, we can be sure we have taken the wrong turning.

The achievements of intelligence therefore also have their pitfalls, even more difficult to identify than the lure of the senses. We are only too ready to admit, "Oh, I can never resist chocolate." But how many of us would admit that we would willingly stab any colleague in the back in order to gain a promotion? We shy away from such self-knowledge as we instinctively feel that its ugliness lies closer to the Soul.

Most of us, at least in maturity, with or without yoga, fall into a dutiful routine, a comprehensive conduct of trying to "be good" and fearing the consequences if we are not. This is neither solution nor resolution, but it is a livable cease fire, or decency by dint of moderation. Controlling our desires is a continual pruning process, rather than a Damascene conversion.

Yama and *niyama* (the ethical code) assist us in this reasoned restraint, acting as a firebreak for our behavior. Asana is a cleansing agent and pranayama begins to tug our consciousness (citta) away from desires and toward judicious awareness (prajna). Pratyahara is the stage at which we learn to reverse the current that flows from mind to senses, so that mind can bend its energies inward. Dharana (concentration) brings purity to intelligence (buddhi), and dhyana (meditation) expunges the stains of ego.

Concentration brings "purity" to intelligence. You must be protesting that throughout this book intelligence has been presented as an unalloyed good. It has received no bad press at all. This is fair enough when you are laboring up the lower slopes of the mountain of yoga. The ascension to lofty intelligence is ardently to be desired. But now we are in the sheath of intelligence itself, the vijnanamaya kosa, and we have to remind ourselves that the five afflictions (klesa) taint every level of our being, except the pristine Soul itself.

We have honed, cultured, and refined our intelligence. We have realized its power to discriminate and choose and its capacity to move us incrementally toward freedom. It is reflexive, so that we can witness ourselves. Exalted, unconditional, pure intelligence is a close and near neighbor to the soul. So why am I sounding a warning that "As the hot coal is covered by smoke, mirror by dust, embryo by the amnion, so the intoxicated intelligence covers the Self" (Bhagavad Gita 3.38), suggesting that even here its imperfections have to be sifted and only the diamonds retained?

High intelligence brings the gift of power, and we all know that power corrupts. When intelligence is corrupted, it brings woe upon ourselves and upon the world. Its impurities reveal themselves in base or mixed motivation, selfish intentions, pride and the pursuit of power, self-seeking ambitions, ill will, calculation and manipulation, hypocrisy, chicanery, cunningness, arrogance, disingenuousness, and secret joy in the discomfiture of others. These impurities stem more from the conative aspect of intelligence (will, volition, intention) and less from its cognitive and reflective side. They contain an instinctual biological distortion, expressing itself as "What's in it for me and mine?" and contempt for others in an "I am right; you are wrong" attitude.

We said that intelligence, by consulting memory, can factor in consequences. What intelligence does not do well is pick up on its own motivations that are quietly infiltrating from ego. To see impurities of intelligence, just buy six different newspapers on the same day or watch several different TV news stations. Notice how the same events come to be reported so differently. This may be simple misperception, but more likely there is a slant or twist of interpretation that serves the agenda of the newspaper proprietors. This may be nationalistic because they have links to a governing party, or it may be a hidden economic interest. After all, most newspaper owners are by definition rich men, bent on getting richer. Notice too what is left out and what is included. We are forced to conclude that the vaunted objectivity of media is too frequently superficial or hypocritical. This is not because the journalists' minds do not function well. They do. It is because there is subversion in their intelligence. These are called impurities, and they are very difficult to detect in ourselves. If we live outwardly virtuous lives, it is easy to convince ourselves that there is nothing else wrong with us. Often this is the besetting sin of the puritan or religious fanatic. In our personal lives, we often both suppress the truth and suggest the false. Ego aids and abets all flaws of intelligence.

These impurities of intelligence are the high crimes of humanity, and we cannot disown them. But we can get rid of them with help from the part of our consciousness that is closest to our soul.

Conscience

Intelligence can be largely self-policing because it has the ability to initiate action and the ability to factor in consequences of these actions. A conscious effort to observe and identify these defects (in ourselves, rather than in others) pays dividends. Such self-examination forms an integral part of the study and education of self (*svadhyaya*), which is the fourth segment of the ethical code of niyama. But still we need both a yogic technique and an independent arbiter. I shall deal with the second first. The function of independent arbiter, the witness of the witness, as it were, is fulfilled by conscience (*antahkarana*). This is the face of the lens of consciousness that faces the soul. It is less likely to be tainted by contact with the world than the outward face of the lens, which is in contact, through the senses, with the world about us. When this facet of consciousness, which we call in English conscience, is flawless, reflecting only the light of the soul, it is known in Sanskrit as the organ of virtue (*dharmendriya*).

Cosmic consciousness can be considered in a way to be the soul of Nature, limitless as the universe, all-embracing. That part of cosmic consciousness that is in us is the individual conscience. It is in closest proximity to the Soul (Purusa), and therefore has a very special relationship with soul. It is the nearest point of contact we experience between the natural world and the spiritual world. For that reason, you could say that conscience is the perception of consequences perceived from the deepest level, that of unity. This is where soul infuses matter, a bridge between Soul and Nature. That is why conscience will only ever tell you one thing, offer one course of action, because it comes out of Oneness. Conscience is consciousness being able to tune in to the promptings of the individual soul (*atma*).

Good advice can come from many sources and may all be useful in its own way, but it leads only to a resolution through analysis and synthesis, which is the brain working. Intuition often manifests as an inner voice, arising from fine and sensitive intelligence. It might tell you not to take a particular job in spite of attractive appearances, or to make a journey that you had not envisaged. It is to be respected, though treated with caution, at least until intelligence has reached the stage of pure wisdom. Intuition transcends rationality and is from the heart.

What then is different about conscience? The difference is that conscience hurts; it causes us pain. We say we are pricked by conscience. Intuition prompts us, causes perhaps some confusion, because we do not know where it is coming from. But conscience hurts. That is because it lies at the heart of the paradox of what it means to be a spiritual being, living in a physical body, in a material world. Conscience tells us to do the harder thing, because it is always pulling us toward Unity, toward Wholeness. Our desires, our selfishness, our intellectual flaws always tug us toward the world of diversity, where we judge issues, muddle through, and try to choose the lesser evil. Conscience, when it is flawless, is the voice of our soul, whispering in our ear. In that sense, even a painful conscience is a privilege as it is proof that God is still talking to us.

This close juxtaposition of conscience and soul reminds me of a visit I made to Rome many years ago. Pope Paul, the then pope, was in poor health and invited me to come and see him with a view to giving him yoga lessons. I accepted. But suddenly, at the behest of his cardinals, he imposed a condition. The lessons were to be kept a total secret as it might be interpreted in a twisted fashion as if a Catholic Pope were to be seen to be following practices associated with Hinduism. Of course, I assured him that yoga is universal, transcending any creed or cult, and I was able to say that I would not broadcast what was taking place. Nevertheless, I said, if questioned about it, I was not prepared to lie. Apparently my truthfulness presented a security risk, and the lessons never took place.

However, I did visit the Sistine Chapel and saw Michelangelo's great ceiling painting of God, reaching from a cloud, extending his finger to Adam, who in return, also extends his hand toward God. Their fingers almost touch. This is what I mean by the relationship of soul to conscience. They almost touch, and at times a divine spark passes from the heavenly outstretched hand to man's.

Dharana—Concentration

I jumped over the yogic technique for purifying intelligence and will present it here as it leads directly to meditation, which is the technique for purifying ego. The journey's end is really not far now, which is why yoga insists, go on, go on, redouble your efforts, renounce the fruits of your progress, the powers and honors you have accumulated. Don't fail now when you are so near. Yoga expresses this sense of both urgency and danger by saying that those who are on the verge of enlightenment will be tempted from the path even by angels. This exists in Christian tradition too. Remember when Jesus was very near to his goal that the dark angel took him into a high place and showed him all the lands of the earth and offered him power and dominion over them. He too was a supreme renunciate, a *bhaktan*.

As I said in chapter 1 Dharana (concentration), Dhyana (meditation), and Samadhi (total absorption or bliss) are a crescendo, *samyama yoga*—the yoga of final integration. Because Dharana is so easy to translate, we often overlook or dismiss its importance. Paying attention in yogic terms is not concentration. True concentration is an unbroken thread of awareness. Yoga is about how the Will, working with intelligence and the self-reflexive consciousness, can free us from the inevitability of the wavering mind and outwardly directed senses.

We said earlier that a chattering mind is a lot of little, distracting waves. Concentration is one big wave. Bring many to one. Subsume the many in the one, then calm the one for meditation. You can't calm many waves. I explained that in an asana we send our attention, which is a wave, to our right knee, left knee, arms, right inner knee, left outer, etc. Gradually, awareness spreads to the whole body. At this moment, our awareness is unified. We have brought all the disparate elements under the control of one flow of intelligence. This is concentration or one powerful thought wave. This is the big thing we learn by learning many little things. A mind that can learn to concentrate in this way, to bring unity out of diversity, can now aspire toward serenity, which is the meditative state where even the big wave of concentration is brought to a state of tranquility. There is no way to circumvent this process. You can't count back from ninety-nine (diversity, multiplicity) to zero (a calm meditative state) without passing through one (concentration).

When each new point has been studied, adjusted, and sustained, one's awareness and concentration will necessarily be simultaneously directed to myriad points so that in effect consciousness itself is diffused evenly throughout the body, a penetrating and enveloping consciousness illuminated by a directed flow of intelligence (subject) and serving as a cognitive and transformative witness to body and mind (object). This is dharana, a sustained flow of concentration leading to an exalted awareness. The ever alert will continually adjust and create a total self-correcting mechanism. In this way, the practice of asana, performed with the involvement of every element of being, awakens, sharpens, and cultures intelligence until it is integrated with senses, mind, memory, and self. Thus the self assumes its natural form, neither bloated nor shrunken. In a perfect asana, performed meditatively and with a sustained current of concentration, the self assumes its perfect form, its integrity being beyond reproach. This is asana performed at the sattvic level, where luminosity infuses the whole pose. It is therefore also a meditative asana. I do not say, "I am meditating." I am not.

I am practicing asana but at a level where the quality is meditative. The totality of being, from core to skin, is experienced. Mind is unruffled, intelligence is awake in heart rather than in head, self is quiescent, and conscious life is in every cell of the body. That is what I mean when I say asana opens up the whole spectrum of yoga's possibilities.

Meditation (*Dhyana*)

I have often said that yoga is meditation, and meditation is yoga. Meditation is the stilling of the movements of consciousness. It is bringing the turbulent sea to a state of flat calm. This calm is not torpid or inert. It is a deep tranquility, pregnant with all the potential of creation. Remember the biblical phrase from Genesis—"And God's breath moved upon the waters." When you ruffle the waters, you create. You create everything in the manifest world, from nuclear war to Mozart's symphonies. The yogi is journeying in the opposite direction, from the world of things and events, which are so joyful, painful, baffling, and unending, back to the point of stillness before the waves were ruffled. This is because he wants to answer the question, "Who am I?" He hopes that if he can find that out, he will be able to answer the questions, "What is my source of Being?" and "Is there a God I can know?"

The culmination of this chapter is the experience of the existence and plenitude of the individual soul. But the practice of meditation extends into the next chapter, which concerns samadhi (total absorption and immersion in the Ocean of Being or Universal Divine). The frontiers we create to explain are artificial. Yoga is a ladder we ascend, but whereas with a real ladder, when you are on the seventh (dhyana) rung, all your weight is on that rung, in yoga your weight is still equally on the preceding rungs that have aided your ascent. Should any one of those crack, you fall. We shall see that especially in chapter 7 when we examine the ethical code that is both the foundation and, in its realization, as you say in English, the proof of the pudding.

Where meditation is concerned, I am a purist. I must be; I am a yogi. That does not mean that there is anything wrong with attending meditation classes to relieve stress and achieve relaxation. It is simply that as a practicing yogi, I have to declare the truth; you cannot meditate from a starting point of stress, or bodily infirmity. Meditation is the Olympic final for yoga. You cannot turn up half fit. All the preceding stages of yoga have served to train you up to tip-top condition.

Yogic meditation is not a benign somnolence or torpor. It is not placidity. A cow is placid, without practicing yoga. Meditation is sattvic—luminous, aware. When it is tinged by placidity or torpor, *tamas* (inertia) has tainted it.

Sympathetic wave patterns or vibrations act as mechanical stimuli to bring the mind under control. I mentioned the calming effects of the waves of the sea and could add the wind rustling the autumn leaves. Regular wave patterns from natural sources have a sedative effect upon the vibrations of the human brain in the same way that if you leave a lot of pendulum clocks in the same room, the pendulums will all swing in harmony, though the timing of the swings may differ. Yoga, however, teaches you how to achieve harmony by yourself, without sympathetic support. The benevolent somnolence that such devices induce are useful for reducing stress when you go to the dentist, which is why they play background music of mountain streams, goats' bells, and waves on the beach. They are pleasant, soporific, and not meditation. What most people call meditation is really better thought of as stress reduction or mindfulness training.

Yoga texts do suggest objects such as beautiful flowers or a divine image as aids to meditation. Yoga also stresses that internal objects of concentration are superior as they carry the attention inward toward the soul. There are various points in the body that are recommended for this, from the tip of the nose inward.

What I suggest is concentration on the breath. Nothing penetrates deeper than breath or is more pervasive. Immediately you will object that the moving breath is like the waves of the sea—constant but moving—therefore not a thorough challenge for dharana. You are right. But what of retention of the breath? Breathing stops. Is not the cessation of the movement of breath, the life-giving force, the greatest point of stillness imaginable? Breath moves; retention does not.

Yogic meditation is performed alone, not in groups. It is not a lonely activity but aloneness like the illuminating moon that can lead to the Ultimate and Transcendent Aloneness. Do not confuse Aloneness with loneliness. Loneliness is separation from the cosmos. Aloneness is to become the common denominator of the Cosmic All. The arrested breath, perceived with the unwavering eye of dharana, bears consciousness to its core. It halts the movement of thought. As Patanjali wrote, *Yoga citta vrtti nirodah*. Yoga is the cessation of the fluctuations of consciousness. I said that dharana purifies intelligence. The still mind is, by definition, pure.

Is this the end? Are we there yet? No. There remains the ego, the self, the known self, the impersonator of the Soul. He is the last actor to leave the stage. He lingers even for the very final hand clap of applause. What forces him off the stage? Silence and retention of the breath.

As we saw in chapter 3, there are essentially two types of retention and of realization. At the full, after inhalation and, on empty, after exhalation. In the process of inhalation it is the Self that comes up as the breath goes in. In retention it is the Self that enfolds the frontier of the body in union with the Self. In this state there is a full experience of Self that is egoless but where the ego remains dormant and ready to re-express itself. After exhalation the sheaths of the self move toward the Self. As the air moves out, these sheaths move in. Here there is a full experience of uniting with the Self in which the ego is absent and its potential for selfish action is expunged. Inhalation is a realization of the totality of Being swelling out from the core toward the periphery. It is the fullest realization of what is implied by being incarnate, spirit made flesh, on this earth. It brings the discovery of the individual soul. It brings awareness of every cell in one's being. From the core of being, the individual soul (jivatman), one has fulfilled the implication of being chosen to be born. It is the experience of all of oneself, from innermost to outermost, from subtlest to grossest. If we are a mansion with hundreds of rooms and corridors, we might say that normally we are always in one room or another. We are in our minds, in our memories, in our senses, in the future, eating so that we are in our stomachs, and thinking so that we are in our heads. We are always in one bit or another, but we never occupy all our inheritance. To experience the totality of being is to be in every room of the mansion at once with light streaming out of every window.

What happens when we retain the breath after exhalation? There is no thought of duration. One does not say, I'll hold it for thirty seconds, or forty. There is no thought. Thought has ceased. Therefore retention is spontaneous.

Yet there remains one issue. From where does the impulse come to retain the breath in the first place? An act of will or a decision is implicit in the fact that one holds the breath at all. This impulse (prerana) can only come from nature, which is, after all, at the intelligent origin of self—self not Soul. So ego must still be, in however shadowy a form, present. We say that dhyana erases the impurities of ego, if not its actual existence. It happens in this way. Just as the cessation of the movement of thought brings purity to intelligence, so a motiveless retention effaces ego. What the practitioner eventually experiences is not that, at some point, he suspends the breath. He is no longer the subject, the agent. The breath breathes him. What this means is that, at the highest level of meditation, the cosmos breathes you. You are passive. No individual or personal will is present, therefore, no ego, no self. In Hindu terminology, it is as though Brahman, the Creator, is expressing himself through you. You are the expression of His will and design, just as the completed canvas is that of the creative artist. The unpremeditated retention of breath after exhalation opens the gap in the curtain of time. No past, no future, no sense of passing present. Only presence. If, in relation to the individual soul, we talked earlier of the cup being full, full of light and being, this is the complementary opposite. The cup is empty, no self or ego, no intention, no desire. It is timeless, divine emptiness. And this is the fusion with the Infinite, called samadhi, which we shall look at in the next chapter. Samadhi is an experience to be gone through. It is not a sustainable or a livable state. We use the word *kaivalya* for the state of Ultimate Freedom that follows samadhi, a state of aloneness, which means that one has merged with the infinite and can therefore never again be taken in by the appearances of the world of diversity.

We shall see how when the cosmos breathes you, rather than the reverse, the object has subsumed, swallowed up the subject, which is an end to duality. The end of duality that comes from meditation is the end of separation and the end of all conflict. The yogi stands one and alone.

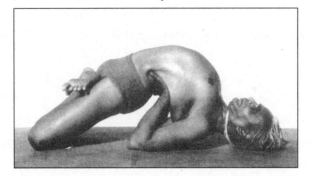

Chapter 6

BLISS
The Divine Body (*Ananda*)

Our Inward Journey has now taken us to the innermost core of our being, to the bliss body or divine body (*anandamaya kosa*) that resides within us all, where our soul lives and where we can glimpse the universal oneness that embraces us all. This vision of our divinity forces us to return once again to the nature of our humanity. Before we can understand the Universal Soul, we must understand our own, and before we understand our soul, we must explore all that eclipses our true selves, especially the wily "I" that takes on a thousand disguises to distract us.

"Who am I?" is a fundamental question that has always existed in people's minds. Traditionally it might have been answered, to some extent, by reference to one's role or primary function in society—I am a priest, a warrior, a merchant, a servant, a carpenter, a wife and mother—but the deeper implications of the question have always been present. In any case, no one is a mother or businessman or schoolteacher all the time, all their lives. These are temporary states. Even if you say, "I am a man, or a woman," it is incomplete. Formerly you were a child, and besides, does sexual identity have any importance when you are asleep?

What we are really saying is "I am I," which is not very helpful. By "I" we are referring to that bit of us that seems to be at the center of our perceptions, our actions, our feelings, our thoughts, and our memories. It is often called the ego-based self, or egoic self. But if all we can say is "I am I," and everyone else is saying the same thing, then logically we must all be the same, which visibly and palpably, we are not. So in order to explain our differences and define this "I" self further, we tack on attributes and characteristics that qualify and exemplify the "I" in some way. A rich man might feel that "I and my possessions" gives a fair indication; a politician, "I and my power;" a chronic invalid, "I and my sickness;" an athlete, "I and my body;" a film star, "I and my beauty;" a professor, "I and my brain;" or a bad-tempered, dissatisfied person, "I and my anger." Adding a ragbag of attributes to our "I" self is not only how we generally see ourselves but how we see and describe others. The important point is that all these qualities we list are external to the "I." In other words, the "I" identifies itself by conjoining with its surroundings.

Clearly I leap-frogged one answer to the "Who am I" question. It is "I am a human being." For this to be of value, one has to ask the follow-up question, "What, then, is a human being?" This is exactly what yoga does. The starting point of yogic inquiry, the basic question underpinning all yogic practice, is simply, "What are we?" Even the asana itself is an inquiry, asking in each asana, "Who am I?" Through the asana, the practitioner throws out all the extraneous parts until only the Soul is left. The final, correct asana is a true expression of "I am That, That is God." This expression is felt only when one approaches and performs asana within the framework of physical prowess (*sakti*), intellectual skillfulness (*yukti*), and devotion and worshipfulness (*bhakti*) in each asana.

Let us therefore sift through everything, says yoga, every component of a human being that we can find and identify—our bodies, breath, energy, sickness and health, brain and anger, and pride in our power and possessions. Above all, yoga says, let us examine this mysterious "I," ever present and conscious of itself, but invisible in the mirror or on any photograph.

The "I" is so often a source of worry. "I" dwells in our bodies, and we know that body dies, brain dies, the heart stops beating, the lungs cease to breathe, and senses no longer feel. Is it therefore not possible, likely even, that the "I" dies too? This is disturbing. If my very identity is transient, ephemeral, what permanence is there? Is there no firm ground? Our lack of certainty is, according to yoga, of itself and by its very nature, toxic. Yoga identifies the very deepest root of all illness as being the sorrow and pain we undergo because we live in ignorance of *purusa* (Universal Soul). Being ignorant of our true Self, we identify only with aspects of the natural world, which is in a state of flux. To identify ourselves, we fix on the aspect of consciousness that dwells in the inner body and is called the ego. There is a great gulf between the acceptance of ego as a necessary alias with which to function in the world and mistaking that alias for our True Self. Inevitably, if we fall for the impersonation of our Soul by our ego, we get caught up in the turbulence of the world around us, its desires, emotional disturbances, afflictions, so-called sins, and ailments or obstacles. Inevitably, I say, because our ego-consciousness is part of that hungry, seeking, insatiable, frantic world. In other words, we have no firm base. We want to be immortal. We know in our hearts that we are. But we throw it all away by misidentifying with all that is perishable and transient.

When we first asked the question, "Who am I?" what we were truly hoping for was to discover an enduring identity, beyond role or function or attribute, a "real" Self, real in the sense that it is not menaced by the mortality of the flesh but that is permanent and unchanging. That is why yoga examines the totality of being, every layer of existence from body inward, sorting, testing, observing, experimenting, dissecting, and classifying until a full blueprint of the human being is built up. The ancient yogis and philosopher saints systematically did this until they found the light they were looking for, the eternal unchanging Self, the part of us that answers once and for all the original, inevitable question, "Who am I?" Their gift to us lies in the knowledge and techniques and maps of their search that they bequeathed to us, so that we too can each answer our own question, since it is certain no one else can answer it for us. In this chapter, we will explore the nature of this eternal, unchanging Self, but before we can, we must discover the Five Afflictions that eclipse our comprehension and cause so much of our suffering.

The ancient yogis tried to work out a plan by which human evolution, both individually and collectively, could progress. In doing so, the ancient sages naturally asked themselves the questions, "What is making things go wrong? Why, in spite of our best intentions, does something always send things awry? Are we programmed forever to sabotage our own aspirations?" Their inquiry led them to the Five Afflictions that we all experience.

The Five Afflictions (*Klesa*)

The Afflictions are a particular pattern of disturbance to the human consciousness, as universal and prevalent as fruit flies to healthy apples. Our state of mind at any given moment is a wave pattern. It is incredibly complex. It is constantly modified by outside stimuli, an advertisement, an unkind word, a smile from a friend. Rising thoughts from the unconscious and memory confuse it further—a wish, a regret. But there are more enduring patterns of interference that I shall explain now. They are as inbuilt in us as fruit flies are in the life cycle of apples. They are called the polluting fluctuations of consciousness or afflictions (*klesa*). They corrupt our lives and vitiate our best intentions to ripen as a person.

There are five afflictions. They are natural, innate, and they afflict us all. The first of them is in effect the father of the other four. If you can overcome it, you will have turned night into day. Whereas certain schools of thought, especially in the West, make an amalgam of all the forces of evil and call it the Devil, yogic thought begs to differ. It too makes an amalgam of all the forces that lead men to perform evil and perverse deeds. The difference is that western thought ascribes the attribute of intelligence to evil. The devil is a clever devil, sophisticated in the arts of corruption and possessing an independent consciousness separate from and antithetical to the aims of man and God. This is a situation of unending conflict between two intelligent and sentient forces, one good and the other evil.

The Devil of yoga is not intelligent. He is ignorant. In fact, he is Ignorance itself. We often think that ignorance means you don't know the capital of Albania. What yoga means by Ignorance can perhaps best be translated as "nescience," which simply means not knowing. So to Hindus, the archenemy is a state of not knowing. What don't we know when we are ignorant?

The answer is this. You don't know what is real and what is not real. You don't know what is enduring and what is perishable. You don't know who you are and who you are not. Your whole world is upside down because you take the artifacts in your living room to be more real than the unity that connects us all, more real than the relations and obligations that unite us all. Perceiving the links and associations that bind the cosmos in a seamless whole is the object of yoga's journey of discovery.

It is this idea that we live in a totally topsy-turvy world that gives rise to the saying that what is day for the ordinary man is night for the wise and vice versa. There is a famous phrase by a metaphysical poet who said that, "A fool who persists in his folly will become wise." The European medieval humanist Erasmus wrote a book called *In Praise of Folly*. From Europe to the Far East, there is a tradition that human perception is so totally flawed that frequently it is the "saintly idiot" who is wiser than all his seemingly sensible neighbors. What this means is that we are not required simply to adjust our vision, but to turn it inside out as well as outside in, a complete reversal. It means that the ultimate truth is inconceivable in normal consciousness.

These statements about Ignorance (in Sanskrit called *avidya*) are challenging. There are various ways to explain them. They are mostly so revolutionary that they require the use of paradox. The Lord Jesus explained it well. He said that if you build a house on sand, it will founder. If you build it on a rock, it will stand firm. This means that a life must be built on a foundation of reality that is firm. Unfortunately, what seems firm, that is to say the things of life that offer us security, wealth, possessions, prejudices, beliefs, privilege, and position, are not solid at all. That refers back to when I said that learning to live with uncertainty is the great art of living. Jesus also means that only a life built on spiritual values (*dharma*) is based firmly in truth and will stand up to the shocks of life.

You could put it this way. All mankind lives unwittingly within the truth of yoga. Yoga is one. No one escapes the mechanism of "As you sow, so shall you reap." Yet we deny the totality of our vision. We find ourselves in the position of having to portion it up, to compartmentalize it, to cherry-pick what suits us and reject what does not. Why? It is because we all misapprehend reality. Not just partially, but totally. Only the supreme renunciate (*bhaktan*) is capable, with one peerless gesture of surrender, of turning the Universe inside out and outside in. In the West this is exemplified by St. Francis of Assisi embracing a leper because he perceived a soul identical to his own within. We others simply cannot. We are like a man who has put his shirt on inside out and back to front. The only way he can rectify his error is to take it off, work out how it should be, and start again. Through yoga, we take off the shirt of our ignorance, study it, and put it back on correctly, as a shirt of knowledge. To do this, we examine (like the man turning out the body and each sleeve of his shirt separately) each petal of yoga as if it were separate. Just as man knows that the shirt is one but has many designs, we should not forget that yoga is only one.

Spiritual values are not the sauce on the dish of material life, perhaps only to be indulged in on Sunday. They are the main dish, that which nourishes and sustains us. Material values are the sauce, and they can help to make life extremely pleasant. In moderation and tasted with detachment, they will make this world a paradise. But they do not endure. Ignorance (avidya) prevents us from seeing the truth—what does *not* endure is the egoic self—ME. The undiscovered soul endures the misperception that *I* am ME. It is this egoic ME that does not want to die. This impersonation of soul by ego is at the base of all human woes, and this is the root of avidya (ignorance or nescience).

Ignorance is, in its essence, taking the day-to-day self we know, for the immortal Self, the true Self or Soul. If you combine that with the fifth affliction, which is Fear of Death and Clinging to Life, it means that a great deal of human activity throughout all ages is an attempt to perpetuate the existence of the ego itself, through name, fame, wealth, glory, or achievement. Yet the soul endures, and the known ego will perish, as does its outward sheath, the body. This is mankind's horrid predicament, that what he believes himself to be, his ego and attributes, are perishable, whereas what man merely senses himself to be, transcendent consciousness and soul, will endure. We cannot endure the loss of the known. We have insufficient faith to place trust in the survival of the unknown. Yoga's answer is to say, "Discover the unknown, and you will encounter your own immortality."

I cannot stress sufficiently that the Five Afflictions are interwoven into the fiber of all our beings. They are not like defects such as laziness or greed, which we may or may not have. They are wave patterns of interference that stem from our glorious individuality, biological, psychological, and spiritual. They are the fundamental misapprehension of the relationship that the part (our individual selves) has in relationship to the Whole (Nature and Divinity). Without a clear appreciation of what we receive from the Whole and what we contribute back to the well-being of the Whole, we are left howling in the wilderness. No lovers, servants, riches, cars, houses, or public acclaim can salve the wound of a dysfunctional relationship with our origin. "Know your Father," said Lord Jesus. By this statement he was directly addressing the problem of not knowing (avidya).

The other four afflictions are the shoots of the root, avidya. The first affliction that emerges from avidya is called Pride (*asmita*). Pride leads to arrogance. Arrogance leads to what the Greeks called "hubris," that is vying with the gods for preeminence. Destruction is the certain result. Yogically all that it means is that the fragile and beautiful stem of individuality that resides in each one of us, pure in origin and intention, meets, as it sprouts, the phenomenon of the external world—clothes, girls, boys, cars, position, titles, money, power, and influence—and subsequently is colored by them. Asmita (I-ness) is pure and colorless, both in origin and when knowledge of wisdom is established. It is purity and singularity without defining attributes. But, as it meets the world, it becomes tainted, colored, by contact, and becomes pride. It assumes the attributes that seem to cluster around it and loses its pristine beauty. That is the beauty we see in a young child, before the world has sullied his or her innocence.

So asmita, our unique and stainless individuality, can, through the saddening and obscure years of life, harden into an exclusive shell of selfishness, of me, of pride. This pride lies in difference, not in equality. You are pretty, but I am ugly. I am fierce, but you are weak. I own a house, but you are a beggar. I am right, but you are wrong. It is, in effect, ignorance (not knowing) raised to the level of a political platform. It is the insanity of individualism, when it should be the joy of singularity. Pride blinds us to the quality of others. We judge by externals and by worthless comparisons. We lose the possibility of joy in the existence of others. We expect others to perform according to our desires and expectations. We are constantly dissatisfied. To borrow a golfing metaphor, we lose the ability to play the ball where it lies.

The first two afflictions, Ignorance (not knowing) and Pride, are considered to be wave patterns of interference operating at an intellectual level. The next two, Attachment (*raga*) and Aversion (*dvesa*), influence us more at an emotional level. We must be careful with language here. When we say, "I am very attached to my wife," we mean, "I love her." So it is only a manner of speaking. What raga really means is obsessive or perverted love, a conflation of the egoic self with the object of one's attachment. We have all witnessed the car owner who, faced with a tiny scratch to the bodywork of his vehicle, leaps from it like a berserk warrior who has received a wound in battle. What we witness here is a fusion and absolute identification between the ego (which does not endure) and an object in its possession (which does not endure either). We all know the phrase concerning death: You can't take it with you. This is true. I cannot take my ego beyond the grave, and I certainly can't take my car, my land, or my bank account. The dominant word here is "my." You can easily see how this is the child of ignorance—one impermanent entity seeking an enduring link with another impermanent entity. It is quite insane from a logical point of view, which is why I said earlier that we must take off the shirt of ignorance and turn it inside out. There is no way to adjust it when you are still wearing it. The word raga therefore applies to the magnetic attraction between ego and the pleasant objects that surround it.

The correct attitude to our "possessions" is gratitude, not ownership. Toward our car we should feel gratitude that it conveys us safely and allows us to see places we would not otherwise have seen. I am grateful to the table I am writing on. It makes this book possible. Whether it is "my" table or not is irrelevant. In India we have a ceremony every year in which we garland our household objects and thank them for the service they render us. We borrow their services for a certain time and are grateful. But the table is a table and will probably still be doing its job long after my death but not indefinitely.

What, you must be asking, is the case when someone you love dies? You are sundered. There is a rending pain of separation. Of course there is. But this is not raga. I lost my wife suddenly, brutally, unexpectedly. I was not even there, but away teaching in Mumbai for the weekend. I could not get back in time. I did not cry at her funeral. My soul loved her soul. This is love. It is transcendental and transcends the separation of death. If my ego, my small self, had been the source of my feelings for her, then I would have cried, and mostly I would have been crying for myself. There is nothing wrong with shedding tears for ones we love, but we must know for whom they are shed— for the loss of those who remain and not for those who have departed. But, as the poet says, "Death shall have no dominion."

Aversion (dvesa) is the opposite side of attachment. It is a repulsion that leads to enmity and hate, like the same poles of two magnets pushing away from each other. Again it is based on superficialities. My essence cannot hate your essence, because they are the same. I may deplore your behavior, but it is a nonsense to deduce that therefore I hate you. If I, on occasion, have deplored my own behavior, does that mean I should hate my own soul, hate the divinity within? Of course not. I should correct my behavior. Again it is ignorance that plays the puppet master and sows confusion. If we conflate what people do with who they are in their deepest origin, we lock ourselves into an adversarial and aggressive crouch, an unending conflict. By doing so, we sign up for a permanent war between good and evil, which cannot be won. All we should seek is for evil-doers to reform their deeds. The best way to help them is to reform our own deeds, and then we may well discover that all mankind is much of a muchness, one essence common to all, and that all our woes stem from the fundamental misperception of ignorance. Ignorance here comes to mean the denial of original oneness or universal community.

The final wave pattern or affliction that influences our lives is experienced at an instinctual level. At an instinctual level, it makes good sense, as we are all animals trying to stay alive. It is when we upgrade a natural survival mechanism to inappropriate levels that trouble arises. It is called Fear of Death or Clinging to Life (*abhinivesa*). Naturally when you are sick, your biological body clings to life; it is supposed to. This is the struggle for existence, the reasonable desire to prolong the life of the vehicle of the soul. After all, it is not like a car. You cannot just buy another one. You have to keep your body as healthy as possible on the spiritual path.

We all identify with our bodies. This is inevitable. If an elephant charges toward us as we cross the road, we do not cry, "My God, my ego will be crushed!" At that moment we are our bodies, which jump out of the way. This is largely true when we are ill. Good health banishes body identification to a degree nothing else can.

We accept that, in the long run, we are not our bodies. Body perishes; we hope we will not. But you cannot tell that to pain. We may know that body is not our enduring identity, but that knowledge is theoretical. In health we forget our bodies; in sickness we cannot. How much simpler life would be if this were the other way round. In relation to the body, this means that we are not our body in any permanent sense, but for all practical purposes we are our bodies, because they are the vehicles through which we perceive and can discover our immortality. This is why yoga begins with the body.

Nevertheless, we accept that body will perish, lamentable though that may be. What we do, however, find intolerable is the fact that "I" shall die, that my ego is as perishable as my flesh. This brings us back to ignorance. Our ego is the most intimate and interior part of ourselves that most of us know. If ego perishes, we fear that we shall be engulfed in darkness, in an everlasting void. So we conclude that we must perpetuate ego at all costs, through dynasties, fame, great buildings, and all immortality projects aimed at cheating the Grim Reaper. What rubbish, says yoga. Ego is an important component of consciousness that you require to operate your body during its life. Beyond that it has no purpose.

But consciousness is much more than our egos. It is even, according to yoga, more than our minds. Scientists are beginning to ask the question, "How does mind give rise to consciousness?" Yoga would ask, "How does consciousness give rise to the mind?" It is its precursor and not limited by the physicality of mind. Consciousness exists at a microcosmic level, i.e. smaller than the atom. According to some scientists, cosmic intelligence exists at a quantum level. Mind, (*manas*) is the most physical and external part of consciousness. Being the most material or manifest, its fortunes are linked to those of the body for good or ill, which is why a car accident can leave you "brain dead" but not consciousness dead. In near death experiences, people retain a form of awareness but without its constituent parts. Even when all neurosystems, including memory, have totally shut down, consciousness continues as a witness, though at a level that cannot yet be scientifically perceived. Because intelligence (*buddhi*) exists in us as a particle of a universal phenomenon, it cannot be totally eclipsed, even when we suffer physical damage. In the same way, soul cannot be killed. Only its vehicle can die.

Look for the light. Ego is not the source of light. Consciousness transmits the divine light of origin, of the soul. But it is like the moon; it reflects the light of the sun. It has no light of its own. Find the sun, says yoga, discover the soul. That is what *Hatha Yoga* means. *Ha* is the sun—the Self; *Tha* is the moon of consciousness. When the lens of consciousness is perfect and clean, it will be clear that its illuminating light is the innermost soul. The soul is divine, nonmaterial, perfect, and eternal. In other words, it does not die. Discover what does not die, and the illusion of death is unmasked. That is the conquest of death. That is why I did not cry for my wife, in spite of all my pain, for I will not cry for an illusion.

Because this affliction concerning the finality of death is necessarily and usefully instructive, it is the hardest to break, even if we grasp it, as I am sure you do, intellectually. We are not required to eradicate it from its appropriate biological sphere, but to repulse its invasion of "nonbiological" realms. The instinctual urge for the body's survival is one thing and very necessary. But we want to go further. We want our genes to live on in our progeny. We want our children to live in the country house our family has lived in for generations. We want our businesses to survive and prosper, even after our retirement or death. We want, if we are artists or scientists, to be enshrined in posterity. When we extend that instinct to survive to subtle areas such as the perpetuation of the ego, it can be psychologically destructive.

THE FIVE AFFLICTIONS ARE SO FUNDAMENTAL to our lives and our ability to navigate the journey of yoga that I will recap them. Avidya (ignorance, lack of knowledge, lack of understanding) is the fundamental misapprehension that material reality is more important than the spiritual one. It is not because all things material are transient, impermanent, and susceptible to constant change in the form of growth and decay. The problem is our dependence on what will not last. When asmita expresses pride, it gets confused. Yet it is an extraordinary gift of individuality with the experiences and material objects that the individual encounters in the course of his life.

Raga (attachment or desire) is an emotional bondage to any source of pleasure, manifesting in extreme forms as an inability to let go of anything, a sort of addiction to the furniture of life rather than a celebration of the joy of life itself. Dvesa (aversion) is an emotional repulsion and flight from pain, manifesting as prejudice and hatred and making it impossible for us to learn from life's hardships and our own mistakes. Abhinivesa (fear of death) is an instinctive clinging to life, which, though appropriate at a biological level, causes perverted attitudes when transferred to aspects of life where it does not apply. Abhinivesa can easily be experienced if you over-prolong the retention at the end of exhalation. Panic sets in. It is ignorance, or the fundamental misapprehension of Reality, that underpins and feeds all the other afflictions. If you want to see the power these afflictions have over our lives and human history in general, just watch the evening news on television and identify these five destructive influences at work. That is easy. Then apply them to yourself.

The Goal Can Be Reached

Meditation is the gateway to ending the Five Afflictions. Meditation is bringing the complex mind to a state of simplicity and innocence but without ignorance. Meditation comes when ego is vanquished. As the seventh petal of yoga, it can be reached by progressing through all other stages of yoga practice. But the eighth petal, *samadhi*, comes as the fruit of meditation. It arrives by the Grace of God and cannot be forced. Samadhi is the state in which the aspirant becomes one with the object of meditation, the Supreme Soul pervading the universe, where there is a feeling of unutterable joy and peace.

In the past chapter, we explored the point at which the totality of being was experienced, from core to periphery, an expansive, creative movement that revealed the individual Self (*jivatman*). The focus of this chapter, the blissful sheath (anandamaya kosa), is the surrender, and fusion, of the individual Self in the Ocean of Being. It is not merely the transcendence of ego but the dissolution of self as we know it, a hiatus in the ongoing experience of self. It brings us to the original illusion (avidya) of separation between Creator and created. It is truth incarnate. It is truth in spirit. It is the divine marriage of Nature and the Universal Soul. It is existential and supra-existential bliss, total absorption in Origin and End. It is to be born to the eternal.

For most of us, now and throughout past history, samadhi remains theoretical. Yet yoga shows the way to this lofty peak. For the vast majority of readers, it is envisageable only as a heavenly landscape of beatitude that we conjure up through imagination (*vikalpa*). Yet do not think for a second that I am saying it is not real or that you cannot reach it. The ultimate freedom is not beyond your grasp. Examine your imagination. Are you daydreaming of the future or trying to remember the face of a long lost love whose features have melted in the mists of time? It is the latter. And does not the longing you feel spring from the core of your being? Is it not a desire for an end to duality, for a Oneness that is not achieved through complementarity, but a Oneness that exists because there is no Other.

To discover the individual soul you need inspiration, the creative force of breathing in. To discover the Cosmic Soul you need the courage to release, to breathe out, to make the ultimate surrender. Do not be discouraged. The Divine Will impels humankind to this end. Hold the soul (*atman*), not just the breath. There is a space between surrender and acceptance. You surrender to the Lord, and the Lord accepts your surrender. And, to accept, time and space are needed. That is retention (*kumbhaka*).

The Final Ascension

I have deliberately given a sneak preview of the majestic crescendo of our quest. This is because there remains much to learn and much literally soul-searching work to be done. I said that we have to apply our observation concerning the afflictions to ourselves. Therefore we need a mirror. So we have to continue our practice of yoga, all aspects of the practice we have learned hitherto. We have to refine what we already can accomplish and add new depth and subtleties in order to penetrate into the final heart of the mystery. We have to keep on questioning ourselves, or else transformation will not take place. Advance with faith, yes, but always call yourself into question. Where there is pride there is always ignorance.

Before our consciousness finally gravitates to our Self and our Self is merged in the Infinite, there are many fine threads to be woven together into the shimmering cloth of our practice. We have to weave in a meditation of such selfless purity that the impersonating ego will be unmasked for all time. When the ego is effaced, the afflictions that accompany it will disappear. Another thread that we must weave in is an understanding of how the elements inform our practice. I have discussed in the earlier chapters the elements of earth, water, fire, and air and how they correspond to the first four sheaths of body, energy, mind, and intellect. The final element that corresponds with the final sheath of bliss is called "space" and allows mobility and freedom in all the others. Space is the most subtle and pervasive element, and we must learn to tame it.

Space, sometimes translated as ether, is not the ether of the modern chemist. It is taken in its old sense as being the space permeating the emptiness between particles of matter. The amount of matter inside an atom is equivalent to a tennis ball inside a Cathedral, so our atoms, and therefore we, are almost entirely space. The spaces above us, the sky, is *mahat-akasha* (cosmic intelligence in space) while the Self within is *cit-akasha* or *chidakasha* (cosmic intelligence inside us). One is the external space, the other is the internal space, but to yogis the felt space of the Self is actually larger than that of the external space surrounding them.

Space is emblematic of freedom, the freedom that only space allows for movement, for is not change itself a movement? The view that astronauts gained from outer space often left them with a unified, nonpartisan, borderless perception of the planet earth that changed their lives and led them to try to impart their experience through the pursuit of shared human goals to be achieved by peaceful cooperation. As I have said, we cannot all go into orbit, but we do have access to space, our inner space. Paradoxically, looking within has a comparable unifying effect as visiting space does for astronauts. I make no excuse for repeating that inside the microcosm of the individual exists the macrocosm of the universe. If this truism, however obvious to you or however unlikely, does not hold good, then all yoga is nonsense, along with Gnostic mysticism, Sufism, Buddhism, and the teachings of Christ.

The wisdom that yoga practice has given me was confirmed through the sacred yogic books that I have read. Not only have I acquired knowledge by my *sadhana* and the reading of sacred texts but also through my travels and the people I have met. All these weave together the last threads of our yogic cloth.

The writers of the Vedas were seers, but also poets and visionaries who saw divinity everywhere, in everything, in animate and inanimate, organic and inorganic things. Somehow we have lost that art. Stagnation has brought insensitivity, but echoes of wisdom persist. The great Catalan architect Gaudi, for example, said that architecture was a creative relationship between the sensuousness of Nature and the austerity of geometry. This is a theme that runs through yoga practice. My attempts systematically to impose symmetry on asana postures express this relationship. And, as with the architect, the concept of space is fundamental. A vase, like a building, like a body, has two spaces—the one that it contains and the one that surrounds it. When we begin asana, we worry about the shape of the pose, that is, how we look in the mirror, in other words, the space we exclude. By now we should be worrying about the space we *include*, the space within, for it is largely that which gives true life and beauty to the asana. It is called *yoga svarupa*—the self assuming its perfect form through yoga. That is achieved through the inner distribution of space. Essentially that is how *yogasana* becomes effortless, with the natural beauty of molten gold being poured from a vat.

To reach the Infinite, we have to use finite means, as does the architect, even if he is building a cathedral or a temple. And, like the architect, yoga science says that you have to align your inner and outer bodies, so that they run parallel and are in communication with each other. Without correct alignment, a building falls down. Gaudi sought to express the sublime through the physical. It is the same for the yoga practitioner. Alignment creates an intercommunicating structure that, like a cathedral, is an offering to God. That is why for me alignment is a metaphysical word. Correct alignment creates correct space, as in a well-constructed building. A building without a spacious interior is a lump of stone—a megalith. Can you imagine a body like that? It would be both inert and uninhabitable.

According to Indian philosophy, art is of two types. One is called *bhogakala*, the art of appeasing the pleasure of the body and mind. The other is *yogakala*, the art of auspicious performance to please the spiritual heart of the soul. All arts have science (*sastra*) and art (*kala*). Bliss (*ananda*) is experienced and expressed when the goal is to bring order out of chaos, wisdom out of ignorance, divinity out of aesthetics. Do you wonder that I become angry when my students throw away their God-given talents on *bhoga yoga*, look good, feel good but do no good yoga?

The drive within Nature is to express itself through evolution. That is especially obvious to anyone living in a tropical country like India. Nature wants to occupy every space. That is mirrored in our language when we say that "Nature abhors a vacuum." Nature sees its role as expressing itself in more and more variety, and often, to our eyes, in more and more beauty, but not always in beauty. Nature can overwhelm us. Why did yogis go to the Himalayas? Was it to find space, an outer space to reflect an inner?

Earlier I related air to touch and to intelligence. I said we both inhale and bathe in it. Space is even more intimate, more pervasive, since all of our atoms are mostly composed of space. Sound and vibration correspond to space and can travel through them like the radio waves that we send out through space in the expectation that intelligence will some day be able to communicate fully. Is sound not even more powerful and more intimate than air? The vibration of a whale's song can penetrate hundreds of miles of ocean. Is not the sound of God (AUM) more holy than any idol? Is not music the highest art? Vibration is a wave. It comes from three points—all that is needed to make a sine curve—and is the first step of manifestation. It is very close to the root of nature, and it is very powerful for that reason. As I have said, "When you collapse your posture, you collapse your soul." When you collapse the space, you collapse the soul.

The eyes are the index of the brain. The ears are the index of consciousness. The eyes belong to mind and fire, the ears to awareness and space. When one is in a meditative state, the frontal brain is resting and without interruption. Whenever we are thinking about a problem, we lean our heads forward. If you let your head drop forward in meditation, the frontal brain will feel distress. But if there is harmony between the eyes and ears, the focusing of awareness becomes easy. The eyes are the window of the brain, the ears are the window of the soul. This is contrary to popular wisdom, but when the senses are withdrawn (*pratyahara*) this is the true experience. The ears are able to discern vibration. Our inner space corresponds to what we normally call Heaven. This is how we can hear the divinity of our inner heaven before we see it. The ears also witness silence. Silence is the music of samadhi.

Let me be more prosaic. Just as we cannot separate the element of earth from the sheath of our physical body (*annamaya kosa*), so we cannot separate space from the blissful sheath (anandamaya kosa). In asana, we are playing with the elements. When we twist, for example, we are squeezing space out of the kidney, and on release, space returns, but space renewed. Similarly, we are squeezing water, fire, and air, as well as to some extent earth, out of an organ when we twist or contract.

When we release, circulation comes back, restoring revitalized elements. We think of this as washing and cleansing the organs. This is true, but at the elemental level, what we are doing is playing with the balance of the elements, experiencing which sensation each will bring us.

In a twist, it is not only the organ that is twisted, but the bones, muscle, fiber, and nerves. The vessels carrying liquid will also be constricted. The mind will take on a different form corresponding to the unusual shape of the body. The intelligence will touch the body in a different way, and the vibration that the body emits will be altered; for example, I am able to feel the vibration of each kidney and to compare the difference between them. This twist will also bring into evidence the subtle qualities or counterparts associated with each element. For example, it will make us aware of the density, strength, and scent of the body's clay; the flexibility and taste of the body's fluids; the vitality and vision of the mind's fire; the clarity and touch of the ambient intelligence of air; and the freedom and inner vibration of the ethereal space within the body.

This is how we learn to discern and appreciate the subtle elements of nature of which we are composed. It is like *lila*, the Sanskrit term for the cosmic game, but played at a very high level. As animals learn the arts of survival by playing when they are cubs and puppies, so for us this game is an essential step in learning how to survive in the subtle heart of nature. It is exploration through play, through trial and error. When we can play with the elements within our own bodies, with their renewal and disproportion and rebalancing, then we are aware of nature at a level that is not apprehendable in a normal way. It is supranatural, as normal consciousness is blind to it. We are discovering evolution through a journey of involution, like a salmon swimming back up the torrent from which he was born to spawn again. We must now look at the evolution of nature itself so that the yogi, like a Himalayan Sherpa, may achieve his final ascension and conquest. Only when he stands on the peak of nature will the yogi meet his soul—Pu-rusa—and also *Purusa-visesa*—the Universal Soul. To stand on it, in truth, is to *understand* it.

The Evolution of Nature

It is worth pointing out that there is no inherent antipathy between Darwinian concepts of evolution and yogic theories. Yoga has faith in the existence of God. But it does not see God as a puppet master, pulling the strings of a trillion marionettes simultaneously. The world as we experience it is connected to and imbued with the reality of Cosmic Soul. But it is not directly manipulated by it. This way of looking at things is entirely in sympathy with yogic attitudes.

Yoga agrees, which is why it is deemed to be a dualistic philos-ophy, Nature on the one hand, Soul on the other. To yoga, nature is na-ture and spirit is spirit. They intercommunicate, and the spiritual Soul is supreme, the abiding reality. But we must take nature seriously as we belong to it and live in it. To dismiss it as an illusion by a philosoph-ical sleight of hand is, to the yogic mind, naïve. To accept visible na-ture as the only reality is ignorance personified. To the yogi, nature is a mountain to be climbed.

Yoga sees the origin of nature as a root. In Sanskrit it calls it root nature, (*mula prakrti*). Within that root, as we saw earlier, exist certain unstable but creative propensities called the qualities of nature, the three *guna*: mass or inertia (*tamas*), dynamism or vibrancy (*rajas*), and luminosity and serenity (*sattva*). In the root of nature, they are bal-anced and in equal proportions. They exist only as a potential. They do, however, partake of nature's enduring characteristic. They are un-stable. They shift. It is their destiny to fidget and form.

And form they do, but gradually. The subtle precedes the gross, or as we would say, the invisible comes before the visible. Cosmic intelligence (*mahat*), which exists in all of us, is the first manifestation of the invisible. From cosmic intelligence sprout cosmic energy (*prana*) and consciousness (*citta*), and from these devolves ego (*ahamkara*) or the sense of self. From the one root comes duality (which is the ability to separate), from duality comes vibration (which is the pulse of life beginning), from vibration comes invisible manifestation, and from the invisible comes the visible in all its glorious and horrendous diversity and multiplicity. This end product is what we take the world to be— our playground, our paradise, or our hell and our prison. If we misapprehend nature, take it at face value, through ignorance (avidya), then it is our prison.

The path modern science has taken to escape from the prison is analytical. Science dissects, whether it be frogs, human bodies, or atoms. It seeks truth in intrinsic minutiae. But if you take a watch to bits, you may understand how it works. However, you will no longer be able to tell the time. Yoga also dissects—ego, mind, and intelligence, for example—but it is not only analytical. It is synthetic too, or integrationist. It examines in order to know, like science, but it wants to know in order to penetrate, to integrate, and to reconstruct through practice and detachment the perfection of nature's original intention. In other words, it wants to reach the root and cut out the intervening turbulence. It does not want to be hoodwinked by nature's appearance, but to adhere to its original motivation.

The difference between yoga and Darwin lies in the theory of natural selection by the random mutation of genes that provides survival advantages on a haphazard basis. If it is the subtle that clothes itself in the form of the gross, this cannot be. Two centuries earlier, Isaac Newton followed the yogic line. He said, "The order that reigns in the material world indicates sufficiently that it has been created by a will that is filled with intelligence." This, clearly, is not the puppet master creator, but an innate natural intelligence seeking to express itself. But do not forget that order and chaos make strange bedfellows, and the results are unpredictable.

Yoga would say that this unpredictable diversity stems from the intelligent will and life force of nature (*prerana*) struggling to express itself in more and more ways, like an actor who wants to take on as many different roles as possible. To yoga, the code embedded in DNA is not some inexorable deterministic force. It is deterministic to the extent that it carries the code of past *karma*. But it is also the will of nature seeking freedom through individualization. To take an example, the particularity of the flounder fish, which has two eyes on one side of its head, lies on the bottom of the sea bed and is dark for camouflage only on one side, is not the result of a freak mutation, but the flounder's response to the challenge of existence in a dangerous world, animated from within and motivated by an unconscious cellular intelligence.

The reason behind our exploration of the elements and their subtle counterparts is to penetrate into the evolving heart of nature, to catch it before it shows up in obvious objects like trees and tables, hotels, saris, and motor cars. Beyond even that lies our wish to reconcile the gunas, the unstable qualities of nature that lend it both its creative and transient characteristics. At a material level, inertia/mass (tamas) predominates, which is why it hurts when you stub your toe on a table leg. At a psycho-sensory level, dynamism (rajas) and luminosity (sattva) are predominant, which is why studying for an exam can be an exhilarating experience, shame over a mean action can be fiery torture, and a job well done can be a source of *sattvic* serenity. The yogi aims to be a *gunatitan*, one who can restore the guna to their original proportions and then draw them all back up in a stable form into the root of nature and so transcend their vicissitudes. Henceforth he is unshaken by the turbulence of nature.

This does not mean you are unfeeling. I referred earlier to the loss of my wife and the fact that I did not cry. Do not think that I did not, and do not still, feel it as much as any man. The yogi is human. In fact, through the compassion he gains, he is the most human of humans. Nevertheless, in the transcendent but razor-alert peace of meditation, he views life from the summit of Mount Nature.

The qualities of nature (guna) have until now been treated as the most arcane of esoteric knowledge, unsuitable for the general public. I do not believe in that attitude. I suffered from it when my own guru said I was unfit for *pranayama*. Yet the subject is difficult, and so for the sake of the general reader, I will offer one last analogy. In all phenomena the three guna are present, but always in variable proportions. As the proportions change, so do natural phenomena emerge (which we call birth), grow and decay (which we call existence or life), and disappear again (which we call death). The odd but striking parallel that I offer you is not supported by scientific knowledge on my part. It is Einstein's famous equation $E = MC^2$, in which E is energy (rajas), M is mass (tamas), and C is the speed of light (sattva). Energy, mass, and light are endlessly bound together in the universe. An analogy of this might be that light itself (sattva) displays in physics dual attributes. It is neither a wave nor a particle, yet, depending on the method of observation used, it can be perceived as either a discrete photon (tamas) with a specific location or as a wave (rajas). Even at our more prosaic level, we can learn to observe the changing interplay of these three properties.

There is a practical point to this. Once the principles of nature have been withdrawn into their root, their potential remains dormant, which is why a person in the state of samadhi *is* but cannot *do*. The outward form of nature has folded up like a bird's wings. If the practitioner does not pursue his practice with sufficient zeal, but rests on his laurels, even at this point, the principles of nature will be reactivated to ill effect. Many are the God-men who have fallen.

Yoga As Involution

We all want to develop and improve ourselves. We think of this as personal evolution, and a spreading of our wings. The true yogic journey is involution, or to refer to the previous paragraph, folding one's wings. If evolution is a preparation for yoga (the intention to unite with the soul), then involution is actual yoga (union itself). We struggle from the gross material world into the subtle heart of nature, like the salmon returning to their source for both death and regeneration. The force that is expressing itself welcomes our journey, even though it seems to obstruct it. So we must do everything we can to encourage our development through asana practice and stopping our self-destructive habits, such as smoking or overeating. We also use our will, (not ego but our nature's life essence) to favor the struggle. And we invoke divine aid in an act of surrender and humility. The combination of these three makes the journey possible.

Let us take two examples, in relation to what I have just said, of how one might attempt to change one's life. Let us imagine a man, short of money and in a dead-end job. He is anxious, stressed, and frustrated and irritable with his wife and children. On Friday nights he tries to escape his predicament by drinking too much. What can he do? What does he do? He makes the effort not to go out drinking. This already is a small victory, but what can he do then with the money he has saved?

He can go and buy a lottery ticket or several. The odds are against him, first because he is behaving weakly—it is his ego that is asking God to let him win—and there is no role for the exertion of his own will. To buy a ticket requires little effort, and there is nothing practical he can do to make his ticket win. The only thing he can do is not lose the ticket. All parts are weak—his divine relationship, his natural life force, and his practical action. This is the feebleness of fantasy and tenuous connections.

Let us say he takes a different course of action. He spends the little money he has saved on an evening course to improve his skills. Ethically he strives to improve his relationship with his wife and children, recognizing that whether the fault is his or not, the solution is in his hands. This is a purifying process and one involving sustained personal effort and sacrifice. He asks God from a humble heart to help him find a better job and endure better the one he has. Nothing happens. Time passes, the economy improves. His new skills are noticed as well as his new maturity at work. He is promoted and has prospects. The strain at home is relieved at every level. This is not a fairy tale. Our man has made valid connections, and he has shown patience and perseverance (*tapas*), physical prowess (sakti), study (*svadhyaya*), intellectual skills (yukti), and devotion (bhakti) in the chosen path. His outward change of fortune expresses a powerful inner change. He has brought Nature and Soul into closer harmony, and the result is what we call success and happiness.

You may be surprised that I use such mundane examples in the samadhi chapter, but do not forget that it is all the eight petals of yoga that form the flower. Perhaps for the man above, his samadhi was a worthwhile career and happy home life. Equally, the highest practitioner who abandons the two petals of the ethical base will fall. So many people approach spiritual growth as if it were a lottery. They hope that some new book or new method, some new insight or teacher will be the lottery ticket that allows them to experience enlightenment. Yoga says no, the knowledge and the effort are all within you. It is as simple and as difficult as learning to discipline our own minds and hearts, our bodies and breath.

Samadhi is ultimately a gift from the divine, but how do we make ourselves worthy to receive this gift? We must return to the subtle, but also to the all-pervasive cosmic energy, breath, (prana). I have mentioned that it is the first form to evolve from cosmic intelligence. The term breath is inadequate to express its scope, its ability to act as the messenger of the gods. According to the Upanishads, it is the principle of life and consciousness. It is even equated with the soul. It is the breath of life in all manifestations of the universe, whether they physically breathe or not. The animate are born through it and live by it, and when they die, their individual breath redissolves into the cosmic breath. Read that sentence again; it is breathtaking. It is survival, not the individual survival our ego craves, but survival and perpetuation nonetheless. Our breath returns to the cosmic wind. The Hebrew of the Bible conveys this same insight, as the individual *ruach* (breath, spirit) is the same word as the cosmic *ruach* (wind, spirit) that in the creation story "hovered over the deep."

Prana, because it evolves directly from cosmic intelligence, carries an ongoing record that is never terminated and cannot be destroyed. I used the simile of the salmon swimming back up the torrent toward its source, as we are trying to do. I said that the current seems to obstruct and oppose us. Prana furnishes us with the fins and flashing tail that enable us to leap the torrent. It, above all in Nature, is attracted toward source, in a parallel sense to the longing of the individual soul for reconciliation with its universal origin.

I was touched and interested to see very recently the humble admission by Stephen Hawking, the great Cambridge astronomer, that he has changed his mind on an important issue. Until now he has claimed that whatever enters a black hole in space can never emerge again, not even light, because the gravitational pull is too strong. Now he says that he has discovered evidence that proves that what he calls "information" does escape from black holes. Prana is the vehicle of cosmic intelligence, which others might call information, and to the yogic way of thinking, Professor Hawking's new view can only seem right. Prana is both being (*sat*) and nonbeing (*asat*). It is the source of knowledge, and in no part of the universe can it be absent or finally imprisoned. Remember that knowledge has a beginning but no end. A black hole is nonbeing, but even that will change again into being. Prana presents us with this paradox. It is the most essential, real, and present feature of every moment of our lives, and yet it remains the most mysterious. How can we reconcile this fact within our practice? How do we relate Professor Hawking's theories on the macrocosm to our practice in the microcosm?

When we are in the suspension of breath in the deepest meditation, a spontaneous, as it were, God-willed retention, we enter the black hole, the vortex of nothingness, the void. Yet somehow we survive. The curtain of time, time that inexorably brings death, is parted. This is a state of nonbeing, but living nonbeing. It is a present devoid of past or future. There is no self, no meditator, no longer even any breather. What comes out of that black hole, that nothingness? Information. What is the information? The truth. What is the truth? Samadhi.

Samadhi

In effect what I have just said is that the mind is a bottomless pit, like a black hole. Stop trying to fill it as it cannot be filled. Go beyond the bottomless pit to realize the soul. For the beginner, samadhi is an alluring subject. But there are reasons not to get fixated on it. The beginner can only conceive of samadhi as a glorification of the self he knows. In the same way, every beginner who picks up a tennis racquet dreams of winning Wimbledon or the U.S. Open. Often beginners in yoga indulge in fantasies of an easy samadhi, and there are those who are only too ready to take advantage of their gullibility.

Samadhi has to come on its own. It is inexpressible. You cannot even ask someone who has been in meditation, "Did you meditate for two hours?" How could he know? It is a state outside time. Meditation is going from the known to the unknown, and then coming back to the known. It is impossible to say I am going to meditate, or I meditated for two hours. If we know it lasted two hours, we were in the self and not in the Infinite where time, in the linear sense, no longer exists. This holds true even more of samadhi. Nobody can say "I am in samadhi." One cannot talk or communicate. Samadhi is an experience where the existence of "I" disappears. Explanation can come only through the presence of "I," so samadhi cannot be explained.

We are now in the innermost sheath, or causal body, where we can see that we are divine and the self with a small "s" is replaced by the big "S" Self, as we truly understand at the core of our being that our individual soul is part of the Universal Soul. It is said that the meaning of life becomes apparent only in the face of death. At this point in practice the ego dissolves, or rather it gives up its impersonation of the true Self. This is the culmination of yoga, samadhi (blissful absorption), the final freedom whereby the individual soul merges in the ocean of being. All this time we have identified ourselves with our bodies, our organs, our senses, our intelligence, and our ego, but here we are totally with the soul. In meditation, consciousness faces the soul itself. Samadhi is seeing the soul face to face. It is not a passive state. It is a dynamic one in which the consciousness remains in a state of equilibrium in all circumstances. The disturbances of the mind and emotions fade away, and we are able to see true reality. Our consciousness, clear of thoughts and emotions, becomes transparent. It becomes crystal clear, as both memory and intelligence are cleansed. As a flawless crystal reflects any color without any blurring or admixture, our consciousness, when it is pure and untainted by disturbances, reflects the object of thought clearly. Whether we look at our work, our marriage, or our children, we do so clearly and, without the clutter of pollution, we are able to see the truth. When the clouds covering the sun move away, the sun shines brilliantly. In the same way when the covering of the self in the form of afflictions, disturbances, and impediments is removed, the Self shines brilliantly in its own glory. After significant effort, a yoga practitioner reaches a state where some asana poses are effortless. What we achieve here externally is achieved through samadhi internally. It is an effortless state, where one experiences the grace of the Self. This is a state of great bliss and fulfillment. Samadhi can be explained by the head, which does not embody the real truth as samadhi can only be experienced by the heart. Few of us may get all the way to samadhi, but we are concerned here with evolution and progressive growth and change. And it is this growth and change, this ever greater ability to see the truth, that will allow us to live increasingly in freedom.

There are problems with samadhi, as there are with every other petal of yoga. For example, if someone asks the question of a saint, "Are you a saint?" there is no truthful answer. As it is an experience out of time and space, without historical record, what is the answer? If a saint says, "Yes, I am," he becomes a non-saint, a liar in that moment, because he is not in samadhi when he replies. He can reply only from his present self. If he replies, "No, I am not," he is a liar too as he has touched the state of samadhi and seen the ultimate reality. It is not a question that can be asked or answered.

As for myself, I am often reluctant to declare that I am a yogi. I can say only that I am on the path, and I'm very near. I can say I'm a forerunner no doubt. I am near the goal, let it come on its own. I have no motive. I had lots of motives in the early days. I have no motive now. My motive is only to continue what I learned so that I may not slip back. It's not an ambition, but I do not want to have a fall—*anavasthitatva*. And I do not want to develop the character of *tamasic* nature in my system, that's all. You may ask, why do you practice then? I practice so that the tamasic nature may not dominate over my sattvic nature. "Renunciation in practice" was my answer to a lot of people who wondered why I continued to practice even after I had achieved what I wanted. But by "renunciation" I mean freedom from the egoic self. When one stops thinking of the "effect" or the fruit, it is a deep, inward experience. It is not meditation as the term is used today, which is a kind of sedative, a drug, which does not allow full spiritual growth. *Dhyana*, yogic meditation, is electrifying. Through it one withdraws from the periphery to the core. This very journey from the periphery to the core is detachment (*vairagya*). There is a detachment from the effect and attachment to the Soul. One has to transcend the *tri-guna*—sattva, rajas, and tamas—while practicing. Only by balancing them to their constituent proportions of one-third each, can they be transcended. At that moment they are reabsorbed into the root of creation, without their inherent instability. Since it is sattva that is most lacking, that is why we place primary importance on its cultivation.

Samadhi is a state of experience where even the existence of "I" disappears. That absence of "I" is a state to be experienced and cannot be explained. But by giving indications on how to live, one can guide the practitioner on the right path. You cannot learn ethics (*yama* and *niyama*) through exercises and techniques. The universal ethical fundamentals of yama and niyama can be explained as they are simply principles to be followed. As beginners we do the best we can, but eventually they have to be applied with full awareness, moment to moment in any situation, under any circumstances. Yama and niyama have to be inspired by example and mature through practice. Asana, pranayama, and pratyahara, withdrawal from the senses, are based on techniques that can be explained, performed before an expert, and therefore corrected. But *dharana*, dhyana, and samadhi are experiencing states, not susceptible to tuition through explanation. In the end, you either reach dharana, dhyana, and samadhi or not. If anybody says, "I am teaching meditation," then, as a student of yoga I say, "It is rubbish," because meditation cannot be taught, it can only be experienced. Relaxation can be taught and is of immense value. If it leads to serenity and well-being, then it is a form of preparation for meditation but should not be confused with the real thing.

I have mentioned that samadhi has its problems. The first is how to conceive of it, as it is unknown, and yet to aspire to it without greed.

The second is that, if you experience it, you cannot explain it, since it is indescribable. If one tries to explain the state of samadhi itself, one should suspect that he has fallen into the trap of dishonesty or self-delusion. The third is that even within samadhi, you can get stuck. Traditionally there is a demarcation of different degrees or qualities of samadhi. I will take them only as two categories. The first group, or lower experiences, are known as *sabija samadhi*. *Sabija* means "with seed." What this means is that although the experience of bliss is felt, the seeds of desire remain in the ego as a future potential. Even after the experience of samadhi, these seeds can sprout again and cause a relapse. The ego has not been entirely purified by the fire of the experience. This particular point on the yogic journey, although so elevated, is one of danger as it can become a wasteland in which the practitioner gets stuck. This state is called *manolaya*, which means an alert, passive state of mind. But in this context, it implies a complacency with what has been achieved and a tendency to slacken efforts to complete the final step of the journey. The yogi cannot rest on his laurels but must press on to the higher states of samadhi in which even the seeds of desire are burnt out from the ego forever and can never sprout or trouble him again. This is known as *nirbija samadhi* (seedless) in which the feeling of bliss is not dependent at all even on a vestigial ego. This is the bliss of the absolute void, of nonbeing transformed into the light of being.

There is a story about this concerning the great nineteenth century Bengali saint Sri Ramakrishna. He was a spiritual genius and from early days slipped easily and unwittingly into a state of (seeded) sabija samadhi. His particular devotion was to the goddess Kali, and in his bliss he was in her presence, in a familiar and divine love. One day a traveling Vedic monk, an ascetic, came by the temple where Ramakrishna was living and questioned him about his experiences. He suggested that Ramakrishna had the potential to go further and so told him to meditate. This Ramakrishna did and slipped into samadhi, a condition that was by now quite natural to him. Then the monk took a shard of broken glass and pressed it between Ramakrishna's eyebrows. Ramakrishna's reaction to this was both terrible and transcendent. In his spiritual ecstasy (inner bliss) he felt himself with a sword kill his consort goddess, the being he loved and worshipped above all. And so he passed into (seedless) nirbija samadhi, the void, the final state of aloneness, a Oneness with no Other, like the pure beauty of a prime number to a mathematician—an indivisible state. It sounds cruel, but at last he was truly and forever free. He had achieved the ultimate goal of yoga.

Lest you think that we are simply in the realm of anecdote and metaphor, I want to express the physical and even neurological basis for the bliss of which we speak. It is the reflective processes arising from the back of the brain that also work to lead us toward the state of bliss that is ananda. The brain stem is the location of asmita, which is the seed of individuality. Above it resides the hypothalamus, which is the neurological nexus of the whole body. Patanjali called this the place of the moon (*chandrasthana* or *anandasthana*), the seat of bliss. It corresponds to the navel, which is the seat of the sun (*suryasthana*). There must be perfect alignment between them for energy to flow uninterruptedly and equally; the four spheres of the brain must be in balance. In this way, the human body acts as a spindle or perfect conductor between the earth and the heaven, linking the two forces that form us through their divine marriage. The lunar plexus keeps our body cool and leads to a cool brain. All pains and pleasures are stored here. It is from this source that one comprehends and lives in the pure and tranquil state of anandamaya kosa, experiencing the core of being.

What Ramakrishna underwent was the final transformation of consciousness. Patanjali described this accession to nirbija samadhi (seedless bliss) in these words, "A new life begins . . . previous impressions are left behind . . . When that new light of wisdom is also relinquished, seedless samadhi dawns."

Yoga describes seven inner transformations of consciousness. They are purely subjective, that is to say, not visible in any external way. They are known only to the practitioner, which is why describing them is rather like describing the colors of the rainbow to the blind. But to give an idea of them, I refer you back to the five objective states of consciousness, right and wrong perception, imagination, sleep, and memory. We know when we are in them and so, to a large extent, do other people. We saw that there is much to be learned from them by defining, refining, and cultivating them. Remember that Patanjali recommended the Healing States of Mind to help us. These also were external or objective and were friendliness, rejoicing in the success of others, compassion towards suffering, and indifference toward the vice of others, all powerful tools that we can cultivate externally by our behavior.

The inner seven states of mind are 1) the observation of emerging thoughts, 2) the ability to nip them in the bud before they occupy and control our minds, 3) the calm and tranquil state that results from that restraint of rising thought, 4) one-pointed attention that is the one great tidal wave of concentration on a given object, 5) the cultivated and refined consciousness that results from this combination of both restraint and power, 6) fissured consciousness, and 7) pure divine consciousness where the practitioner is alone and at one with all.

Any reasonable person must be asking, "Why is the sixth state, almost the most elevated, defined as fissured consciousness, surely a negative or pejorative description?" One-pointed consciousness is like the two edges of the blade. If one is proud of one's achievement, one can be intoxicated by success and then cracks open up in consciousness and asmita is tainted. But if one crosses to the other side, consciousness remains pure and a state of divinity is reached. This is nothing more than the dangerous crossroads of manolaya, in which the consciousness, through the potential of ego to revive and restore itself, retains its inherent flaws and fault lines. From the exterior they will be invisible, but until the final dissolution of ego's presence, they lurk, ready to be reactivated under stress or temptation. That is why only seedless samadhi leads to the final solution of self, the final realization of Self, and the ultimate freedom from the snares of mortal incarnation.

A trivial example of the still slightly imperfect consciousness (*chidra citta*) might be that when, as occasionally occurs, I am invited to conferences with the holy men of India and indeed from around the world, we all stay in a hotel. I cannot help but notice that many of these holy men are unduly and vastly interested to see who has been given which room, who has the most luxurious room with the best view. It is a sort of hierarchical competition for status. One should not make too much of this, but to my mind, it smacks of something short of perfection and humility.

That is why my practice remains unabated. To offer a simile that brings us back to earth, imagine a tennis star, glorious in the prowess of his youthful excellence. Yoga talks of karma (action), *jnana* (knowledge), and bhakti (devotion). These are three intertwined limbs of yoga. The youthful tennis star is engaged in action, winning tournaments, performing prodigious feats as I myself was deemed to do as a young yoga practitioner. I was a star on stage, a marvel of gymnastic ability. Am I now? I am eighty-six years old. Karma and action for me were also always teaching, teaching and transmitting what I knew when I knew it. But the body loses its edge. In 1979 I had an accident that robbed me of my prowess, like the player who damages his arm or back. So I had to learn wisdom, wisdom through adversity. What came back was maturity, an intelligence that informed action, like the tennis star who lacks half a yard of speed on the court, but has learned the subtlety of his craft. What was instinctive had become conscious. That was like a sports star in his waning days, both lesser and greater. But there comes a time when the great tennis champion must retire. He cannot beat the young men forever. He loves the game that offered him a life. Perhaps for years he plays in seniors' tournaments. Perhaps he coaches as well to pass on what he knows to future generations in the hope they will outstrip him. He remains faithful to the game and to its traditions and continued well-being. This is bhakti, service and devotion. For the yogi there is no retirement. But, as for the tennis player, there is a change of state, a role both more humble and more exalted. Maybe the tennis player will one day stop. The yogi cannot. Within the physical limits imposed by age, with a lifelong discipline behind him, and with growing love and compassion, he must continue. He does not want a flawed consciousness. He aspires to the goal, the pure unfissured self, which can never fall back, betray, do disservice, speak untruth, or act meanly or selfishly. The yogi is engaged in a game with no end, for the game is simply the sight of his own Soul.

There has been in recent years a lot of talk about *kundalini*, the yogic life force that lies at the base of the spine and that when aroused and sent to the head can trigger enlightenment. Often it is described as if it were a firework to be set off with spectacular effects comparable to a Fourth of July celebration or the Diwali celebrations. Do not forget that all fireworks come with strict warnings as they are dangerous. You can get badly scarred or worse. Patanjali speaks of the abundant flow of energy in a yogi. Previously it was known as fire (*agni*). Later it came to be called kundalini as the central spinal nerve is *kundalakara*, coiled three and a half times. The awakening of kundalini comes with the divine union of body and soul. Like samadhi, it cannot be forced. It is the power of nature (*prakrti sakti*) that unites with the power of Universal Soul (*purusa sakti*). This creates a huge force that needs inner storehouses in which it can be stocked. These storehouses are known as *cakra*, and in them the confluence of physical, mental, intellectual, spiritual, cosmic, and divine energies takes place. Through the practice of yoga, the flow of these forms of energy can be traced in the visible and invisible bodies and in the known and unknown channels that transpierce our whole body and are known as *nadi*. Kundalini is cognate to the experience of samadhi; it is not a shortcut, a mechanical device that can be activated in order to circumvent the long effort of integration of the five sheaths of body to soul.

I can assure you that everyone seeks samadhi, and most of us seek shortcuts to get there. Those of you modestly struggling to join your hands behind your back (as well as round your knee!) after several years of practice of twistings, may well exclaim, "What can samadhi possibly have to do with me?" Well, for a start, from early chapters, you will have understood that penetration is possible in any asana that you can perform with reasonable proficiency. You may well be going further inside yourself with a few good asanas you can do rather than the one next to you in class, who can do forty with apparent ease. That does not mean we should not strive continually to extend our range. A musical composer may not play every instrument in the orchestra perfectly, but if he wants to write a symphony, he must get to grips with the potential of each one; he must find what it can contribute to the whole, from the French horn to the humble triangle. We have a triangle pose in yoga (*Trikonasana*), and I assure you that when I lost everything in my physical practice in 1979 due to a severe accident, relearning Trikonasana, from the soles of my feet up, made me a master of teaching it in a way I never was before.

What do I mean when I say "everyone seeks samadhi"? Not just through yoga, the slow, sure, safe, and proven method. People seek samadhi through drugs, alcohol, the danger of extreme sports, the romanticism of music, the beauty of nature, and the passion of sexuality. There are a thousand ways, and they all involve the transcendence of the suffering ego in a blissful fusion with an entity much greater than ourselves. When we shed a tear for the two lovers united at the end of a film, or for a character reformed and redeemed, we are expressing our own longing to flee the confines of self, to unite with the greater, to discover through loss of the known, the endless, gorgeous horizon of the unknown.

Some methods of escape are obviously harmful and unsustainable, like drugs or alcohol. Great art, great music, or great works of literature can also begin the work of transformation in the heart of humankind. But I can honestly teach only from what I know. Asana was my school and university, pranayama was where I earned my doctorate, and it is these yoga practices that I have learned for the path to the blissful fusion. Change leads to disappointment if it is not sustained. Transformation is sustained change, and it is achieved through practice. The vehicle of bliss must be strong, especially its nervous system. The highest bliss transforms permanently. Lesser dreams of divine union, however high their aspirations, contain an element of fantasy. They may not be sustainable. We must have spiritual aspiration not spiritual pretension. We may find that the stage on which we strut contains trap doors through which we may fall, like careless actors. Remember the Greek root meaning for actor is "hypocrite." Yoga is solid. It is the path I know, the path I trod, the path I teach. Everyone desires relief from both the restrictions of personality and its impermanence. Everyone desires samadhi. From the dawn of his history, man has sought dangerous, shoddy shortcuts as well as noble ones. Call the hard, sustained progress of yoga a "long cut" if you will, but if it is a long cut, then so is the flight of an arrow.

The final integration of the sheaths of being at last brings access to the knowledge of the soul to join that of the heart and body. Samadhi is only a state where you experience the absorption of the body, mind, and soul as a single unit. But from samadhi, we have to reach a higher and subtler state called *kaivalya* (eternal emancipation or freedom in action). I said that in samadhi you *are* but cannot *do*. What is the condition, following samadhi, in which we can *do* again, but not as before, acting out of diversity and apparent choice? Can I act out of an undivided Self? Can my conscious mind surrender to that which is ever stable and steady? Samadhi, if it was genuine, should have revealed a human intelligence that uncovers the true reality of interconnectivity between people that stems from wisdom as opposed to the power to control people in a way that comes simply from mental knowledge. The person who has that wisdom, and their interactions with the world, are based on a different understanding, one founded in compassion and the friendship of both perceived and realized unity. Kaivalya is samadhi in action, and the subject of the next chapter is how we live with our illumination in the everyday world.

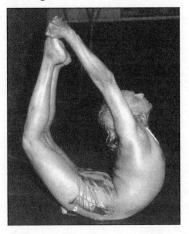

Chapter 7

Living in Freedom

When many of us think of freedom, we believe that it means the pursuit of happiness. Certainly political freedom, as Gandhiji knew, is essential, as the ability to direct our lives is essential for our ability to reach our full potential. Economic freedom is also important, for grinding poverty makes it difficult to think of the life of the spirit. But equally important to political and economic freedom is spiritual freedom. Spiritual freedom actually requires greater self-control and the ability to direct our lives in the right direction. This is the Ultimate Freedom, which is the fusion of our individual soul with the Universal Soul, as we release our own wants and wishes for a higher purpose and a higher knowledge of the will of the Absolute in our lives.

This final chapter on Living in Freedom corresponds to the fourth and final chapter of Patanjali's great work. He calls it the *Kaivalya*

Pada—the Freedom Chapter. Actually he begins his book with *Samadhi*, and then in the second chapter drops right back down to basics, showing how to put one's first foot on the path of the inward journey through the sheaths of being. In his third chapter, he brings us back up to the zenith of yoga but warns of the dangers on the way if we succumb to the temptations of growing power. His last chapter is the most beautiful and lyrical, enjoying the sweetness of the great task accomplished, yet at the same time, he goes out of his way to set our feet back firmly on the ground.

Samadhi is an experience, which he makes clear is worth struggling to reach. It is transformative and utterly purifying. But what then? Samadhi is a state of being in which you cannot do. You cannot catch a bus when in samadhi. In a state of oneness, how would you be able to discriminate which one to get on? Samadhi leaves the practitioner changed forever, but he still has to get dressed in the morning, eat breakfast, and answer his correspondence. Nature does not simply disappear once and for all. It is simply that the realized yogi is never again unaware of the true relationship between Nature and Cosmic Soul. Ordinary people say, "I live my life." The yogi is aware that it is the Divine Breath that lives us. And he can see that Divine Breath in others. His insight penetrates at all times beneath the surface of appearances. Essence is more real than expression.

Kaivalya is both freedom and aloneness, but as I said, it is the aloneness of a prime number that, indivisible by any other number except Oneness itself, lives in unassailable innocence and virtue. The yogi has experienced the freedom that comes from realizing that life has nothing to do with perpetuating the existence of our mortal selves, either in its physical or egoic forms. The yogi has taken the opportunity to encounter the imperishable Self, before all that is transient disappears, as it will, just as a snake sloughs off its old skin.

The realized yogi continues to function and act in the world, but in a way that is free. It is free from the desires of motivation and free from the desire of the fruit or rewards of action. The yogi is utterly disinterested but paradoxically full of the engagement of compassion. He is *in* the world but not *of* it. The yogi is beyond cause and effect, action and reaction. Later we shall see the role that Time plays in this—how there is freedom because the illusion of Time no longer exists to bind us to past and future and so distorts the perfect present.

The challenge for the spiritually free man is to live according to five qualities: courage, vitality, right and useful memory, awareness through living in the present moment, and total absorption in his activities. Spiritual maturity exists when there is no difference between thought itself and the action that accompanies it. If there is a discrepancy between the two, then one is practicing self-deception and projecting a false image of oneself. If I am asked to give a demonstration before an audience, there is bound to be an element of artistic pride in my presentation. But alone, I practice with humbleness and devotion. If one can prevent the inevitable egotism from entering the core of one's life and activities, it means one is a spiritual man. In this state, regardless of the mind, intelligence, and consciousness, he is led from the illuminative wisdom of the core to live a righteous life. He lives from his heart in truth and then expresses it in words.

A spiritual man with his knowledge and wisdom perceives the differences of age and intelligence between himself and others, but he never loses sight of the fact that the inner being is identical. Even though the man possesses an inner knowledge of such depth and subtlety that he visibly lives in a state of exalted wisdom, he also visibly lives with his feet planted firmly on the ground. He is practical and deals with people and their problems as and where they are.

The free man is both innovative and open, even revolutionary, as I have been in my yoga practice, but he will also be steeped in tradition, through culture and heredity. The yogi is rooted in his own experiences and the discoveries he has made through yoga practice. Yet he must continue with an open mind to catch the subtle discoveries that flash up in the *sadhana* and use them to further his inner development. While the yogi is grounded in traditional ethics, texts on the science of yoga, and scripture, he has his own authority as a free man. By free, I mean one whose practices have followed the path of detachment and renunciation to their conclusion that is the unconditioned freedom of kaivalya.

For the average practitioner, remember that learning to live in freedom is a progressive process, as we free ourselves from the habits of body, emotions, and mind. As we gain greater skill, we must always be mindful of how to use our growing power ethically.

Power

Authority brings power, but the practice of detachment reins in that power, preventing its abuse. The power of psychological insight that the yogi gains, his ability to "read" people, should be dedicated to their help and evolution. There is a phrase "Knowledge is power," which is commonly used to sell newspapers and periodicals. Implicit in that sentiment is the belief that knowledge brings power *over others*, whereas the yogi's knowledge is introspective and brings power *over himself*. Allied to discrimination and compassion, that power can be a force for good in the world. The knowledge that devolves from mental cleverness or dexterity, if it is devoid of discrimination and compassion, is heavy with unforeseen consequences. In the case of Faust, he sold his soul to the Devil to obtain this power of knowledge. A clever person may discover a cure for malaria or invent a new strain of anthrax for use in biological warfare. The former obviously possesses discrimination, the latter neither wisdom nor compassion. This is cleverness, the power of the brain, inebriated with itself. Patanjali called the incidental powers that accrue to the yoga practitioner *siddhis*. He was very severe in cautioning against their abuse. He said these powers should be taken as a sign that we are on the right path and then should be ignored completely. Otherwise, they can become traps that ensnare us in vanity and arrogance.

The yogi is by definition beyond such self-intoxication. A yogi's actions may each be very small, but if each is perfect in its time and place, their cumulative effect is considerable. And because a yogi's actions are grounded in example, not precept or preaching, there is a snowball effect by which his actions are emulated by others and passed on with compound interest. This snowball effect that arises from action that is both genuine and disinterested is expressed in the biblical injunction, "Do unto others as you would have them do unto you." Each action is a perfect and discrete module, free of unintended knock-on effects. Even with good intentions, clever people never quite know where they are going. The discovery of penicillin saved hundreds of thousands of people from suffering or even death from, for example, sexual diseases. But even today we all know that sexual license is not free from consequences. My point is not a moral one. It is that what we call "good" in the world of normal causality can quickly change to what we call "bad." The free man, on the other hand, although he still lives in a world of cause and effect, has learned to tread very lightly and to act with great precision.

Cleverness then, acting alone, can be seen as a centrifugal force, likely to spin ever faster and to lose control of its original intention. Yogic knowledge is, on the contrary, a centripetal force, forever discarding the irrelevant in order to invest in the search for the core of being where enduring truth resides. For a yoga practitioner, intelligence is not self-aggrandizing, but it acts like a scalpel, cutting away all that is unreal so that the real and permanent will be revealed. This leads us directly to an examination of the most difficult asana and to the dimension that mankind has not yet integrated in his consciousness: Time.

Savasana and Time

Many people wonder why, in my book *Light on Yoga*, I consider *Savasana* (corpse pose) as the most difficult pose. To most of us, corpse pose is an agreeable payoff after a hard yoga class, in which we feel a relaxation that is either torpid or vibrant or, to some extent, luminous. Luminous here means *sattvic,* which is both aware and passive. Torpid means *tamasic,* and as many of my students come to class after a hard day at work, I have never objected to that. It is only natural, and many snores have provided the music that ends a class filled with even my most senior students. I may be a martinet when you are on your feet, but I do not think I have ever woken a student from Savasana, except possibly in time to send him home. But Savasana is not about falling asleep. If it were, Savasana would hardly be a difficult pose.

Savasana is about shedding, in the same way that I earlier mentioned the snake sloughing off its skin to emerge glossy and resplendent in its renewed colors. We have many skins, sheaths, thoughts, prejudices, preconceptions, ideas, memories, and projects for the future. Savasana is a shedding of all these skins, to see how glossy and gorgeous, serene and aware is the beautiful rainbow-colored snake who lies within. We even lie on the ground as a snake does, with the maximum possible surface of our bodies in contact with the earth.

Now, Savasana is about relaxation, but what prevents relaxation? Tension. Tension results from clutching tightly to life—and in turn being held by the myriad invisible threads that tie us to the known world, the known "I," and the known environment in which it operates. It is the threads that bind the "I" to its environmental context that give us our sense of identity. My students, as they lie on the floor at the end of a hard class, are still aware that they are husbands or wives, maybe still with shopping to do on the way home, with parents waiting for them there, or children who will want help with their homework. My students are tired because they are aware they are businessmen or women who have had a taxing day at the office. Perhaps the day went well—perhaps not. My students are all sons, daughters, husbands, wives, workers, parents, male, or female. A thousand threads of identity bind them to the floor as they lie in Savasana, like Gulliver imprisoned by the threads of the midget Lilliputians.

Savasana uses techniques of relaxation to cut the threads. The result of this is not, as in meditation, freedom, but loss of identity. I do not say loss of false identity because in the world in which we function, these identities are real. Yet taking the long view, they are unreal. Even the fact of being male or female is an identity that can be put down.

To relax is to cut tension. To cut tension is to cut the threads that bind us to identity. To lose identity is to find out who we are not. Did I not say that intelligence is the scalpel that cuts away the unreal to leave only the truth? As you are lying on the earth in Savasana, do you not, when the posture is harmonious and balanced, feel both present and formless? When you feel present yet formless, do you not feel an absence of specific identity? You are there, but who is there? No one. Only present awareness without movement and time is there. Present awareness is the disappearance of time in human consciousness.

The problem with Time is this. We can conceive of it only in spatial terms, like a running river or a piece of string. We divide up the string into decades, years, months, days, hours, minutes, and seconds. These are *lengths* of time, and whatever time is, it is not fair or accurate to treat it as a dimension of space, something to be measured by length, like a wall or a bookshelf. Another problem is that we consider time to be empty, devoid of meaning, like an empty bucket unless we fill it up with something, our activities for example. Whatever else time is, it must be fully realized in and of itself, in its own nature, like a flower growing in the desert that needs no observer to fulfill the potential of its own beauty. If you try to imagine time without using spatial concepts, you will find it extremely difficult. That is why I say we have not yet integrated time in our consciousness, as we have done with the three dimensions of space. The power of science is the proof of our ability to project ourselves in space. But space without time is like muscle without brain.

Time appears to us to move, to flow, and to have duration, length; therefore to be spatial. In other words, we are caught in the apparent movement of time. Yet all spiritual paths talk of the primordial importance of living in the present. So what is the present moment? Is it a second? Or something smaller? Logically, the present can only be an infinitesimally small unit of time, that is to say a second divided by infinity. There is no such thing. As a length of time, the present simply does not exist. How then can we live in the present? It is a paradoxical impossibility.

We have to find the present by other means. The only way to do this is to divorce it from past and future. In that way, time cannot flow. Literally it stops, as it does in meditation or samadhi. Savasana is the key to this understanding. All our identities, our affiliations link us to past and future. Nothing at all in our lives links us to the present except the state of *being*. Acting takes place over time; it has duration. Being transcends time. A state of being can be achieved only by cutting all threads that bind to past or future. I was born a man; I will be a man tomorrow. Can I now, in Savasana, put down even the sexual identity that links me to past and future? Can I exist in a discrete awareness of time in which neither past nor future impinge or taint the present? Savasana is being without was, being without will be. It is being without anyone who *is*. Is it any wonder that it is the most difficult asana and the door to nondualist meditation and the cosmic fusion of samadhi?

When past and future are discarded, what remains must be the present. Suppose you spend five minutes in the present in a wonderful Savasana. Is it a five minute Savasana? No. It is an infinity of present moments, discrete and juxtaposed, but not joined or continuous. It is like looking at a roll of cinematographic film, in which you can see that each photograph shows a picture and then there is a jump, however slight, to the next reality. They do not slide together unless you watch them in movement, when they appear continuous. The psychological flow of time ties us to past and future identities and events. As long as we are caught in the flow of time as a sequence of movements, we cannot fully be in the present. Therefore we live in a sort of compromised reality. That is why I say that time seen as movement and not as presence is an illusion that limits our freedom. Savasana frees us from this. I said that in meditation we open the gap in the curtain of time. It is in Savasana, by becoming nobody, literally nothing and nobody, that we become small enough to pass through the infinitesimally small crack in the curtain. A practitioner who can put aside his every identity can access places where no plump ego could squeeze through.

If skeptics seek an analogy for the seeming continuity or seamlessness of what appears to us a flow of change, you should look at the phenomenon of water heating. It does not get a little bit hotter gradually as it seems to us. Like the individual slides in our film, it jumps. Very small jumps, of course, but water being heated is first one temperature, and then it jumps to another, slightly hotter. There is no between. What this suggests is that life is a series of discrete transformations. We are in one state—we practice, we detach—then we are in another. What we experience as growth or evolution is in fact a long series of little jumps. These jumps are instantaneous, which means they exist outside time as we conceive it. The ultimate yogic triumph is to live in kaivalya, outside time, you might say, but really inside it, inside its heart, disconnected from past and from future. That is to live always in the kernel of the present. It is the integration of the true nature of time in consciousness, and Savasana is the key. By all means, relax, go to sleep even; we are all human, but in Savasana you are on the edge of a great mystery, and if Savasana is the most difficult of all postures, at least it has the saving grace that we can all lie on the floor as we attempt it.

All models for spiritual life or personal growth seduce us into the belief that we are *becoming*, rather than just being. Being is not static, but like the heating water we just mentioned, it is a moment in present time, in a certain state or condition, and from which, if we continue to add the flame of zealous practice, like a Bunsen burner under a retort, suddenly another state will spontaneously emerge, as if by magical transformation. We perceive only the sequence of these transformations in time, which is why we are caught in the illusion of becoming, instead of just being, and then being again, and being again, separately but transformatively, ad infinitum, like the stills of an old silent film, until the story reaches its conclusion and, hopefully, its happy ending.

This idea of a ladder to be climbed, even if it is in some ways flawed and certainly leads to invidious comparisons between practitioners or the establishment of a hierarchy of excellence, is pretty universal. Yoga avoids this because all petals are practiced simultaneously and form a composite whole.

I believe in the perfection of the yogic system as a vehicle to enlightenment. I also support the Indian cricket team. Life puts us in one place and time, and we must live it to the best of our abilities from that point. But when people evoke to me the perennial wisdom of the mysterious orient as if all other men throughout history had been misguided and unevolved, I become impatient. The mind of man is one. The mechanics of consciousness are the same everywhere. A good person, living ethically with his eyes on the stars and his or her feet set on the path of duty is a good person anywhere. A problem is a problem anywhere. To the extent that yoga offers both understanding and a blueprint for action, it offers them everywhere, to all people, at all times. Yoga cannot be preached about, or proselytized. It can only be adopted, and its success in being adopted around the world is proof not of cunning salesmanship but of practical efficacy and high aspirations, which are the province of all humankind.

In order to begin to live in freedom, we must see how this allows us to fulfill the Four Aims of Life throughout the Four Stages of Life.

The Four Aims of Life (*Purusartha*)

Patanjali made it clear in his penultimate verse (*sutra*) that enlightenment and freedom come to one who has lived life fully. Fully and completely—but not excessively or addictively. You cannot rise to the pinnacle of Mount Nature if you are caught up in the excesses of the world. But you can't turn your back on them either. When I was young, as I mentioned at the beginning of the book, I was offered the chance to become a renunciate, a *sannyasin* clothed in saffron. I refused and chose the world. But I did not try to swallow the world, merely to live in it and belong fully to it, passing through the various stages of growth that it offers us all.

The four aims of life that Patanjali said must be accomplished are *dharma, artha, kama,* and *moksa.* These can be translated as doing one's duty by living in the right way (dharma is commonly understood as religion or religious duty), the self-reliance of earning one's own living (artha), the pleasures of love and human enjoyment (kama), and freedom (moksa). These four fit together in a particular way. Otherwise our lives would be anarchic.

Imagine the situation like a river flowing between two banks that control its course. One bank is dharma, the science of religion, or as I consider it, the righteous duty that upholds, sustains, and supports our humanity. By religious I mean the observance of universal or ethical principles, not limited by culture, time, or place. The other bank of the river is moksa, freedom. By moksa I do not mean some fanciful concept of future liberation, but acting with detachment in all the little things of here and now—not taking the biggest slice of cake onto one's own plate, not getting angry because one cannot control the actions and words of those around us.

The river of love, pleasure, prosperity, and wealth flows between these guiding banks. Personal love, part of which is sexual, is a wonderful apprenticeship to love of the Divine. By learning to love one woman, we can learn to love all womanhood, the whole female principle. You simply cannot love your wife and at the same time hate all other women. That does not mean womanhood is a feast to be consumed by one man. On the contrary, the particular is the gateway to the universal. Parents, and particularly mothers, learn to embrace the whole of humanity through the love of their children. I said that I refused sannyasin because I wanted to live in the world with all its turbulence and challenges. I also said that I did not want to swallow the whole world. That is the madness of addiction. You cannot consume the infinite. All you can do is taste its essence through the particular. Dharma and moksa come to our help here.

I mentioned early on in the book how, when I was a young man away teaching for long periods, sometimes female students took a fancy to me. I invoked dharma to sustain and protect me from overflowing the riverbanks of propriety by cultivating a fierce and forbidding manner. Like a reverse magnet, it kept people at a distance and saved me from sliding into easy expressions of intimacy.

On my travels there were other kinds of enjoyment on offer, beautiful landscapes and stimulating and interesting films and theatre. I enjoyed them to the full, as Patanjali intended us to, but the detachment of moksa gave me objectivity. Whatever I saw and learned was considered in the light of "How does this relate to yoga's understanding of the world? How can I use what I am learning to further my practice and teaching?"

In human love I was blessed with a perfect partner, and the river of love ran smoothly. Artha, earning a living, was another matter—whitewater rafting down a dangerous torrent. As a young man I sometimes starved—no money meant no food. I married before I was in a stable situation, and then children started to arrive. I worked flat out,

I borrowed, but money remained a huge source of anxiety. The richest students are not necessarily the quickest or best payers as any teacher will tell you, and I sometimes let myself be exploited. Even when I built my own Yoga Institute in the mid-seventies, problems persisted. There was food on the table, thank goodness, but buildings develop structural faults; governments make tax demands. It is really only just recently that this current of the river has run smooth for me. I live as simply as ever, eat the same, only, with age, considerably less, but I no longer need to worry, and whatever surplus there is can go to projects for schools and irrigation in the village of Bellur, where I was born and that I left in 1925.

Eventually, however, I can say that I have fulfilled artha, raised a family and built a home through my efforts as a yoga teacher. I always had faith, and I always got by, but it was for so many years a very tough ride. I suppose I could have courted rich sponsors and become a parasite as some "holy" men do. But that is not artha, it is not dharma, it is not moksa, and I can only thank again my forbidding manner that kept people at a distance and prevented my river from flooding its banks. Financial security is essential. My experience is that God will take care of you if you have full faith in Him and surrender to him completely.

One way to sum up the four aims of life would be to say that provided you behave ethically on the one hand, surrender to God on the other, between these two, you will Love, Labor, and Laugh.

I have suggested that moksa is a thousand little freedoms that we accomplish each day—the ice cream returned to the freezer or the bitter retort left unsaid. It is our training for the greatest detachment that leads to the ultimate freedom, kaivalya. But if kaivalya is majestic and permanent, we must not belittle the small daily victories of moksa. They come from the persistent and sustained will to be ever more free, to cut the myriad threads that bind us and of which we talked in relation to tension and bondage in Savasana. Anything, however small, that restricts our freedom to act, that is to act from source, from our core, is a cause of tension and stress. Freedom is gained incrementally and over time.

We must return to the subject of Dharma. If we translate it as "the science of religious duty," it immediately raises the question, "Is dharma following the dictates of some religious creed?" Most definitely not. Dharma is not about denomination or cult. It is universal. The second question that arises is, "Is dharma then about being a moral person?" I would reply that what we call moral values are susceptible to change over time and according to culture, place, and circumstance. Dharma is rather about the search for enduring ethical principles, about the cultivation of right behavior in physical, moral, mental, psychological, and spiritual dimensions. This behavior must always relate to the growth of the individual with the goal of realizing the Soul. If it does not, if it is culturally limited or warped, then it falls short of the definition of dharma. Sadhana, the practitioner's inward journey, admits of no barriers between individuals, cultures, races, or creeds. So neither can dharma. The discovery of the Universal Soul through the realization of individual soul is an experience that, by definition, can leave no frontiers intact. I do not object to the word religion—I am used to it—but some people do. So let us just remember that the earliest Latin root of the word religion—*relegere*—means to be aware, and absolute awareness will never perceive difference or conflict. Only partial awareness can do that. Most religious people are therefore only partially religious. That implies that however good their intentions, they still need an even fuller, more inclusive awareness.

I have always been and shall remain an ethical man. The spiritual life I have led has come by the grace of God, but to stick to ethics is our human duty. If we follow certain universal principles in life, God looks after us at all times, smoothing our path and helping us through the hard times. My yoga is founded in ethics, but I must admit I am bred and trained for the ethical life as a racehorse is trained for speed.

Not that my life has always been spotless, but a driving impulse toward ethical integrity is there. It is the plinth on which my asanas stand; it is the rock to defend like a Maharajah defending his hill fortress.

I admit I am steeped in tradition, born of my forebears and transmitted by them. Yet at the same time, I have been revolutionary. I have examined the tradition in order to find the original way of seeing it, to discover its essential meaning by hammering away at it with my own awareness and intelligence. Tradition is like a beautiful statue, which over the years, gradually returns to just a raw lump of stone. It is our duty to chisel away at it and recarve the beauty of the original form within. That is what I have done and why I can say I am a revolutionary seeking to uncover the pristine traditions. I am both original and derivative, new and old. As I have pursued the Four Aims of Life, I have also pursued the Four Stages of Life. And so must we all.

The Four Stages of Life (*Ashrama*)

The four aims of life are closely related to what we describe as the four stages of life (*ashrama*). These are very simple, natural tendencies that we can all experience if we are blessed with sufficient years. One can think of them as supportive shelters that help us to fulfill the four aims of life and keep the river flowing between its protective banks.

The first stage takes us through childhood and adolescence to the brink of adulthood. It is a period when we need to go to school and learn what the people of the world think, even if their conception of the world may be wrong sometimes. It is a time for assimilating traditional knowledge through parents and teachers and elders. It is a time for submitting to a discipline (like going to school to learn mathematics), which we neither always enjoy nor see the point of. This time is known as *brahmacaryasrama*. The word *brahmacarya* suggests self-control, discipline, and continence, and at this point of our lives, wisdom consists of being patient and kind and respectful to our seniors and tutors, even if we cannot really grasp much value in what they are trying to impart to us. At least some of what they say will later declare itself to be of importance in life, and we will be glad we did not reject it out of hand. This is gentle guidance of childhood's energies and not a brutal bridling and suppression of them. Later on, in our own modified forms, we will find ourselves passing on these traditions ourselves, and the important thing is that as adults we should try to embody and exemplify them.

There is also the question of energy. Children have so much. It is a torrent that can break its banks and dissipate itself in self-destructive ways. What the better type of adult and tutor is trying to do is build up the bank of dharma, of sensible, responsible duty so that the torrent of our youthful exuberance should not lose itself in the desert sands.

That is why parents try to restrain sexual precocity, or prevent our staying out too late with other young acquaintances who may embody our worst tendencies rather than our better aspirations. That is why our elders try to rein in the precocious desire to sample the excesses of the world. It is a premature waste of energy. Children have brilliant minds; they can learn computing and math, Latin and Sanskrit as no adult can. If all adolescence is cast away on girl or boy friends for whom one feels attraction but no depth of love, one is wasting one's natural talents. Continence in every sense is not repression. It is directed channeling for a more mature and glorious flow that will come in its good time.

The second stage of life is designated as *grhasthasrama*, and it is the time for earning one's living and sampling the pleasures of the world. *Grh* means house, and so you are a householder with your own roof, a certain liberty, and a spouse to lie beside you at night. The horrors of creeping off to school with a satchel full of books and perhaps homework undone are replaced by the joys of family life. These involve getting up in the night when your babies cry and a bleary-eyed drive to work to satisfy a boss you are sure undervalues you. It involves worrying about rent or mortgage or the children catching a fever, as well as occasional incompatibilities with your spouse. It involves the car you longed for as an adolescent breaking down on the highway. I am not really painting a gloomy picture just to depress you. All I'm saying is that it is a mixed bag. One uses the skills that one learned in the first stage. For me it was a great joy and one I espoused consciously, rejecting the life of the renunciate, the monk, the *swami*. In addition to the joys of returning from travels and successes to my wife and children, there were tough, worrying times too. In other words, to be a householder, though one has access to wealth and sensual pleasures, can be very hard work.

It would be impossible to maintain the day-to-day grind of that work without the science of duty, of dharma, imbibed in the first stage (ashrama) of our lives. For a start we would have no yardstick to compare our hardships and joys with those of other people, of untold past generations. Such ancient shared traditional wisdom helps to keep us going. We have learned human empathy. As one philosopher said in a treatise on the metaphysical basis of morals, "Behaving morally toward other people requires that we respect them for themselves, instead of using them as a means for our enrichment or glory." Without that guiding bank of religious (in the sense that all religions seek self-knowledge) obligation, the householder's life would quickly descend into an inferno of greed and dissension.

Remember the other containing bank of the river of life that flows abundantly with wealth and sensual pleasure is moksa—freedom, but daily freedom in the form of detachment, hard-won in the teeth of life's setbacks and disappointments. Freedom to a child often means the liberty to eat ice cream until he is sick or to stay up watching television till midnight. To an adolescent, it is the rebellious urge to reject the injunctions of his parents and tutors. Rebellion has its place; I have described myself as a rebel, but there is a form of self-destructive rebelling that is a sort of cursed cross-grainedness and unwillingness either to listen (if not obey) or to cooperate within the bounds of family life and politic society. Later on we find that the comity of nations, that is the friendship between peoples of different countries, cultures, and political systems, is founded on that bedrock of tolerant cooperation. It is the bedrock of world peace.

This stage helps in civilizing us by cultivating love, forgiveness, affection, compassion, tolerance, and patience to accommodate the differing emotional and social environments. It all depends upon generosity, hospitality, and give and take. Hence, it is the highest of the ashramas, or stages.

Moksa to a youth is taught as detachment from the vagaries and disappointments of life. To a young child it is explaining that a promised trip to the zoo or amusement park must be postponed because it is pouring with rain. It is explaining that Daddy and Mommy cannot always afford the most expensive toys. Later on it is consoling an adolescent who fails to be admitted to the university of his or her dreams. Sometimes detachment is being willing to concede to our juniors that even adults are fallible and can be wrong—do wrong—and having the humility to apologize. This is the bank of moksa, the training in detaching ourselves from the sufferings of everyday life, in a thousand ways. Often we have to acknowledge those sufferings in order to detach ourselves from them. Conversely, as we all enjoy a thousand successes, having the modesty to share them and "give away the grandeur," that is to say, not to take the glory to ourselves, to our own ego, but humbly to dedicate our fortune to a greater and higher source, to see ourselves as instruments and beneficiaries of fortune but not ultimately as their architect. This is moksa, the sweet, flower-scented, but sometimes sad bank of the river that channels the current of our lives.

The performance of duty becomes instinctive. Detachment is always a struggle. That is why the third stage of life is one of progressive letting go. It is called *vanaprasthasrama*, which means the beginnings of nonattachment whilst continuing to live within the bosom of one's family. To a businessman it might imply turning over the reins of his business to his sons and daughters so that they can fully enter into the householder stage. It is a letting go of control, not of oneself, far from it, but from the minute control of one's immediate environment, of all that one believes one has built up in the world. If the ego is over-dominant, it is letting go of the confusion of who one is with what one has created, a business empire, a civil service department, the smartest, bravest regiment in the army. Your successors will certainly do things differently from you, and it is more than probable that you will not like it; you will feel aggrieved, a sense of loss, even loss of self and self-worth. The third stage of life is gradually coming to terms with that. After all, the clock is ticking, and old age will not be delayed for long, and death will one day come knocking at your door. Best to prepare oneself in time.

Yet unlike retirement in the West, which is just an end to produc-tive work, this is a spiritual stage filled with growth and learning. It is a stage when this detachment allows us to live ever more loosely in re-lationship to our ego. During this stage, we can more easily let go of the identity that we have clung to and that has hindered us on our In-ward Journey. Now we can move further within as we let go of what has tethered us to that which is without. I help in the medical classes at my Institute, but otherwise, over the years, my children and certain students have taken over. I remain there in the background to help with difficult cases and to offer my experience. Others can teach the regular classes, but the medical classes are where my years of exploring every inch of the skin, fiber, and organs of the body are most needed.

Since the death of my wife, Ramamani, thirty years ago, God chose me to be a sannyasin, a state I had rejected as a young man. This is the fourth and final stage of life, one of ultimate detachment, freedom, purity, and readiness for death. Traditionally, even man and wife might separate and go their different ways into the forest to meet their Maker alone and as naked souls. This is no longer the way. There are no longer enough forests, and besides, modern medicine has convinced us that we can cheat death forever in however debilitated a condition. But the yogi meets death as a servant, a warrior, and a saint. He continues to serve God by his devotion and actions; he steps toward death fearlessly like a soldier who would be ashamed to cling to life, and like a saint because he is already part of the Oneness that he has recognized as the Supreme Reality. The yogi cannot be afraid to die, because he has brought life to every cell of his body. We are afraid to die, because we are afraid we have not lived. The yogi has lived.

This is how the aims of life that must be accomplished marry naturally with the evolution of the human life cycle. There is an Indian blessing, "Grandfather dies, father dies, son dies." This blessing means that the natural cycle of life has not been interrupted by calamity and has allowed each one to fulfill his destiny.

Everything I have said has been about living life to the full, enjoying and transcending nature, and encountering the Divine within. All this exists on an ethical foundation, it exists within ethics, and ethical perfection is the only true proof of its thorough accomplishment. One's spiritual growth is only ever demonstrated by one's actions in the world. The first two petals of yoga are *yama* and *niyama*, the Universal and Personal Ethical Code, which I touched on in earlier chapters. We must return to them now in full, because it is here that they guide us as we try to live with ever greater freedom.

Ethics: Universal and Personal

As we have seen, for the yogi, spirit and nature are not separate. The evolution—or involution—that we have achieved in discovering our soul must now be made manifest in our bodies and lives. In fact, one cannot grow spiritually without increasing one's moral and ethical awareness. Progressively we have to transform ourselves in such a way that we can engage and act in the world without becoming entangled and tainted by it.

This refers back to something mentioned very early in the book. For average people there are three types of action, white (sattvic), black (tamasic), and grey (*rajasic*). They bring respectively good, bad, or mixed consequences. But, as we have seen, consequences cannot indefinitely be controlled, and even good actions can end up over time with mixed or bad results. Most actions are grey as we have partially selfish motives and so consequences are immediately mitigated by either our own impurity of intention or our ineffectiveness in carrying out our actions. A yogi, a *gunatitan*, who has transcended the three qualities of nature (*guna*), is able to act in a totally neutral way. He does not seek the fruit of his action to be recognized as virtuous. He remains free from the dualities of virtue and vice, good or bad, honor or dishonor. He becomes a *dharmi*—a righteous person who merely enacts his duty as an end and fulfillment in itself. This is what keeps him clean and free from worldly entanglements. But, as I said earlier, detachment is an ongoing struggle, and the yogi cannot rest on his laurels, abandon his practice, and fall back into the lazy, spoiled habits of a sort of spiritual Maharajah.

Yama is the code of ethical conduct that helps in our behavior toward ourselves and the environment inside as well as outside. Yama is the foundation of yoga. The principles of yama are essential to evolution at every level. Yama being the foundation, its principles are also the structural pillars that support the whole edifice of yoga as far as the roof, which is no roof at all but the infinite celestial vault above.

Now that we have learned to tidy the house of the self and have discovered divinity residing within it, how do we live differently? D.T. Suzuki, the great Japanese sage, said that the ordinary person floats two meters above the ground. The yogi has both feet on the ground. I would suggest the image that one foot is on the earth, whereas the other stands in divinity, but a divinity that is not divorced from practical reality. It is simply that the divine foot lives in Oneness. The planetary foot can handle diversity, the complexity of seeming contradiction.

Yoga means, as in its English derivative, to yoke, to join, to harness, to unite, to bring together. It means elevating the body's intelligence to the level of the mind and then yoking both to unite with the soul. The body is the planet earth in all its diversity. Soul is the spirit, heaven above. Yoga as an instrument joins these, the Many into One.

Ethics is the glue that binds earth to Heaven. One cannot serve two masters. The only way a human being can reconcile the paradox of the demands of earth and soul is through the observation of ethical principles.

Before going into specific details about yama and niyama, it should be said that whereas morals are flexible and culturally determined according to time and place, ethics arise out of the human need to respect the unity of our unique origin and the divine fusion of our ultimate end. At the same time, they make it possible to live convivially in a world in which difference describes reality. Consequently, when ethics and social comity break down, conflict enters most relationships, whether in marriage, in families, or between tribes, nations, ideologies, or cultures. We think that love should obviate the need for ethics, but while it certainly helps, in any negotiation of human needs there will always be a need for ethics. The yogic perspective of underlying unity, of original sameness, supports this logic. From the perspective of underlying similarity, at every level of evolution, it is cooperation, not conflict, that incarnates the higher truth and that serves the Absolute.

Ethics are a human endeavor and, as in sport, the more sportsmanlike we are, the more we raise the level of the game and bring it closer to our highest aspirations. Cheats always lose. They are unmasked because they are transparently dishonest, deceive themselves, and fail in their human duty. The attempt to live ethically brings us closer to our fellow man and to God above. There are no shortcuts, and certainly cheating always brings about its own downfall, as it exiles us from our own soul. Ethics are a compromise solution by which we aspire for the best, but realistically we are aware that everyone does not play by the same rules

Yoga makes a sincere practitioner into an integrated personality. Ethical living aids the harmonious development of body and mind. It develops a feeling of oneness between man and nature, between man and man, and between man and his Maker, thus permitting the experience of a feeling of identity with the spirit that pervades all creation. So it is that action mirrors a man's personality better than his words. The yogi has learned the art of dedication in all his actions to the Lord, and so he reflects the Divinity within him. Integration depends on integrity, and without it fragmentation will occur. I have mentioned earlier that our conscience faces our soul and therefore reflects its truth. To draw closer to one's soul is also to live more and more by the dictates of one's conscience.

Ethics are designed to make life bearable. They are not the dictates of an authoritarian God, but principles based on an Absolute capable of reconciling the One with the Many. In fact, it is better not to believe in God and act as though He existed, than to believe in Him and act as though He did not exist.

Ethics is philosophy in action from giving a customer the right change to not wasting food. No spiritual improvement is attainable without an ethical framework. In yoga it is not a question of acceptance of God or not. Normally, when we question anyone about whether he believes in God or not, we reduce God to a material thing. We reduce Him to the level of matter, to some*thing* that can be believed in. Therefore it becomes a matter of belief. As the Universe, which is beyond the reach of our consciousness, is unknown to us, so the entity that is "God," which is beyond the reach of our consciousness, is unknown to us. God is felt but cannot be expressed in words. Patanjali's description of God is one who is free from afflictions as well as from actions and reactions. He is the supreme *purusa* (*Purusa Visesa*), a special quality that humans have to know. He is ever pure and clean and remains like this forever.

To believe in God, we need to believe in ourselves first. Our consciousness, the *citta*, has limitations. We need to open the horizon of consciousness to see the other entity, "God." Patanjali knew our weaknesses, that our consciousness is caught in fluctuations of mind (*vrtti*) and inherent afflictions (*klesa*). Therefore, we, in general, and in our consciousness in particular, cannot conceive God. If consciousness can be purified, then the existence of the Cosmic Force can be felt. As one increasingly feels the existence and pull of the Divine, one's actions more easily align with the ethical impulse of the Absolute.

Yama: Living with True Ethics

True ethics are not absorbed from outside conditioning. The innate goodness of a horse, for example, or a dog, derives from its nature, although some training and guidance are necessary especially during youth. Morality and ethics come from inside ourselves and are a reflection of consciousness. However these get distorted by contact with society. This disturbs the consciousness (citta) as well as the conscience (*antahkarana*), which, as we have seen, dwells next to the soul and perceives the world as One and not as a battle for survival through the most brutish aspects of our nature. Yoga trains us away from our selfish, brutal motives and shows us how to complete our responsibilities. This is like a hinge where you educate yourself to accomplish an inner transformation from self-seeking pleasures toward emancipation, from bondage to the world to freedom of the Self, from evolution toward the power of knowledge to involution toward the wisdom of the heart and soul. This striving for self-culture is the onset of true religiousness and the cessation of religion as a denomination or rigid pattern of belief. Spirituality is not playacting at being holy but the inner passion and urge for Self-realization and the need to find the ultimate purpose of our existence. Yama is the culture of self-restraint. Through Patanjali's principles of yama, he showed us how to overcome our human psychological and emotional weaknesses. Yama also means God of death. If the principles of yama are not followed, we deliberately act as murderers of the soul. As beginners we may try to control only our bad habits. But, as time progresses, the dictates of yama become impulses of the heart.

The first injunction of yama is not-harming, nonviolence (*ahimsa*) and the second is truthfulness (*satya*). I join these together because they demonstrate how any perfected petal of yoga modifies the whole. Yoga is one, whether you are doing triangle pose (*Trikonasana*) or telling the truth. Gandhiji, the great man of my century, freed India and changed the world by his perfection in the two petals of nonviolence and truth. His nonviolence both disarmed the overwhelming power of the British and largely disarmed the inherent anger and pent-up violence of the subjugated Indian population. He managed to achieve this because both his words and actions were founded in truth. Truth is an absolute of staggering power. The Vedas say that nothing that is not founded in truth can bear fruit or bring a good result. Truth is the soul communicating with the conscience. If the conscience transmits this to consciousness and then turns it into action, it is as if our acts become divine, because there is no interruption between the vision of the soul and the execution of its acts.

Gandhiji reached this point and proved its magnificent effectiveness. But, of course, most of us struggle along in a world of relativity, of compromise, of self-deception and subtle evasion. As yoga practice develops and the afflictions and obstacles to yoga interfere with us less, we begin to have some inkling of the glory of truth. The shame of violence, of harming others, is simply that it is an offence against underlying unity and therefore a crime against truth. Nevertheless it should be pointed out that Gandhiji's extreme austerities, such as his prolonged fasts, were a form of violence (*himsa*) against himself, by which he woke up the world to what people were doing to each other.

Many are the holy men and women who have come to remind of our unity even in our diversity. Ramanujacharya was a great devotee of Vishnu in the tenth or eleventh century who called upon humanity regardless of the boundaries of color, race, gender, or caste to experience divinity, by initiating them with the *bija mantra "Aum Namo Narayanaya."* This seemingly simple "seed prayer" broke down divisions between people by making them aware that the relation of each person with God is equal. It merely means "Blessed is the Lord Narayana" (which is one of the names of God). Centuries later it was Mahatma Ghandiji who united India as one human race in observing truth and nonviolence, the two sub petals of the yama of yoga.

We should not use truth as a club with which to beat other people. Morality is not about looking at other people and finding them inferior to ourselves. Truth has got to be tempered with social grace. We are all guilty of complimenting someone on a new dress or sari because they are so obviously proud of it. Maybe if we had reached absolute truth we would not do that, but in a relative world, of which we are imperfect observers, we occasionally make concessions. I have a longtime student who, without ever lying, always seeks the positive in the people she meets and tries to put a human face on their shortcomings. This is the sympathy that derives from knowing that she once had great faults and feels compassion for those who are still struggling. So she emphasizes their positive potential and does not drive people into the ground for their inherent negative capabilities. Call it looking on the bright side if you will, but it helps to bring out the best in others. Truth is not a weapon to be abused, and the sword of truth has two edges so be careful. The exercise of the yamas, which are the external moralities, can therefore not exceed the culture and refinement of the person concerned. That is, if I pretend to a morality that is higher or greater than I am in fact myself capable of, then I am posing; I am acting hypocritically. So at each stage of our lives, we do our best with yamas, the external moralities, but it is only through refining the self that we really improve the quality of this morality. One hopes that at later stages of one's life, although one has striven all one's life to tell the truth or not to be possessive of other people's property or not to steal, there will be deeper and subtler meanings to these moral principles, which reveal themselves as we progress. They will be more refined within us. So, for example, when we're young, stealing might mean actually stealing something from a shop. Whereas when we're older, we might refrain even from saying a harsh word that might steal somebody's reputation from them because if you destroy somebody's reputation, you're stealing from them. So there are different levels of subtlety, and it is only through finding ourselves that we actually become worthy of the expression of the higher levels of morality. It's not something where we can punch above our weight. We have got to be up to the weight.

Similarly, we cannot impose our truth on others, and we must always make sure that our actions do not do violence to others. Let me give you a mundane example. If I give up chocolate for a year, it is an austerity practiced on myself, a harshness that may lead to better health. If I force my whole family to abandon chocolate for a year, it is a violence practiced on them and is more likely to lead to family resentment and strife than to harmony, whatever the beneficial effect on their health. Once again, example is all, and when example expresses truth, it has the power to transform others.

Non-stealing, or not misappropriating what rightly belongs to others (*asteya*), is the third yama. As children, we learn not to take or steal others toys, but non-stealing has many other implications. Do we not steal when we consume more than our share? Is it not stealing that a small portion of the world's population consumes the vast majority of its resources? And as I suggested just before, there are even subtler

ways of depriving others of what is rightfully theirs—honor and reputation for example.

Before I deal with the fourth yama, continence, I will say a word
on the fifth, which links to the third, non-stealing. The fifth is non-
covetousness, modesty of life (*aparigrahah*). It means living without excess and obviously the two ideas contained there are that one's own
excess might lead to deprivation for another and that excess is in itself
a corrupting force. It leads to the bondage of sensuality and a desire
through possessions to expand the ego. It is me, me, me by means of
my, my, my. If that is your attitude, the Inward Journey is reduced to
farce from its outset. That does not imply that the creation of wealth
is an evil in itself, simply that we must not hoard it like a miser. Wealth
that is not redistributed will stagnate and poison us. Wealth is energy,
and energy is intended to circulate. Look at your car. How much electrical energy is stored in the battery? Not much, just enough to start it
in the morning and switch on the headlights. If the car is just left in the
garage, the battery runs down and the energy is dissipated. But when
the car moves, it generates great energy, replenishes the battery and
fulfils all the needs of the car to function, including the heater, air-
conditioner, windshield wipers, and radio. Energy needs to flow, or its
source withers. By covetousness or miserly clinging on, we stop energy
from flowing, from creating more energy, and eventually, by this offence
against a natural law, it is we who are impoverished and poisoned by
our own hoarding of life's riches.

I come lastly to the fourth yama, continence or celibacy (brahmacarya), because it raises such strong reactions among the public. To most
people, brahmacarya simply means that if you want to be a spiritual
person then you should be permanently celibate. However, since it would
presumably be a good thing if the whole world wanted to become spiritual, we would soon have a planet populated only by dogs and cats and
cows. If God has intentions, I cannot believe that this is one of them.

Sexual self-control is something else. I always wanted a wife and family. I also wanted to be a yogi. In all Indian tradition there has been no contradiction here. When my wife was alive, my brahmacarya was expressed in my fidelity to her. After her death, desire withered, and my brahmacarya has been that of a celibate. I followed truth (satya) during the first volume of my life, and I followed it in the second. Because both were founded in truth and integrity, both bore fruit.

Sexual love, as I have said, can be the apprenticeship to universal love. What would I have achieved in my life without the love, support, and companionship of Ramamani? Probably not much. I was continent, which means I contained myself. Between what? Between the banks of the river of life, one being ethical and religious duty (dharma), the other being freedom (moksa). If the current of my life had overflowed either bank, my inability to control myself, what we call unbridled lust, would have led to loss of the quest for Self. I would have offended against truth and virtue as I conceive them. My wounded conscience would have obscured my soul.

Everyone, however, does not set off on the path from the source point. Many newcomers or neophytes on the yogic path are not disciplined. Realistically I cannot demand it of them any more than I could put them in *Hanumanasana* in their first lesson. I keep on giving guidance. I correct them in asana and try to arouse the principles of yama and niyama in asana. I try to lead them on to higher practice, but this does not happen instantly. Eventually, however, they come to understand that a lack of self-discipline in any area is a waste of energy. For example, even throwing food away is an offence against the life force of the food. If, on the other hand, you overeat, it is an offence against your own life force. Unethical behavior of any sort will not disturb the beginner at all, but its effect at the spiritual level will be highly damaging. If we look at sex only as a moral issue, we will rebel against it. Yama is not a question of just invoking the opposite of what we desire to do, but of cultivating right perception in order to examine the true facts and consequences of the issue we are confronted with.

Yama is the cultivation of the positive within us, not merely a suppression of what we consider to be its diabolical opposite. If we consider the nonpractice of yama in this way, we will be doomed, not to encourage the good, but to ricochet between extremes of vice and virtue, which will cause us nothing but pain and which have no beneficial evolutionary effect on the world. Cultivate the positive, abjure the negative. Little by little, one will arrive.

To refer back to the Shakespeare quote of chapter 3, I would merely say that love is an investment, lust a waste. That is what he means. Lust leads to isolation and loneliness, a spiritual desert. Brahmacarya implies self-containment, the ability to control oneself, either in respect to others or to experience wholeness in asana. It is not abstinence from sexual activity. It is the ethical control of a powerful natural force. The degree of control will depend on the degree of evolution of the practitioner. Continence and constancy are the key concepts, and let us not forget that the root of celibacy in Latin means being unmarried; it does not imply immorality.

Yama can be learned through the practice of asana. Let me give an example of this. If you are acting over-aggressively in one side of your body, you are murdering (himsa) the cells on that side. By restoring energy to the weaker, passive side, you are learning to balance violence and nonviolence. When the shape of the asana expresses the shape of the self, without forcing, deception, or distortion, then you have learned truth (satya) in asana. Be sure that all these ethical lessons can, if you wish, leave the classroom with you and enrich your life. When a practitioner feels in asana that his intelligence is flooding his whole body throughout the sheaths, he experiences a self-contained wholeness, an integrity of being. He feels himself rise above outer attachments. That is the quality of celibacy in action.

Even the deepest rooted of the afflictions (klesa) can be mastered through observation in asana. It is clinging to life (*abhinivesa*). Even the wisest of people are attached to life as it is physical and instinctual.

But letting go at the moment of death is important for whatever may follow after. By letting go, we also release the latent imprints (*samskara*) of this life and give ourselves a clean start in whatever is to come. The integrated practice of asana brings the wisdom that diminishes the ambition for self-preservation. The sublimation of abhinivesa frees the spiritual aspirant from the obstacle of fear. In this way, at the moment of death, we keep our presence of mind. This helps. There is no panic, no hanging on to the past, no fear of the unknown future. Gandhiji, for example, as he lay dying after being shot by a fanatic, kept the presence of mind to call continually on the name of God, Rama, Rama. That is a clean end and a fresh beginning.

The code of yama should stem from the core of our being and radiate outward. Otherwise it is merely a hotchpotch of cultural mannerisms. Niyama addresses directly and immediately the problems of our internal environment. If yama is the root of yoga, niyama (personal ethics) is the trunk that builds up physical and mental strength for self realization. These observances take us from having a bath to meeting God. That is why it is possible to say that yama and niyama are the foundation, the pillars, and the culmination and proof of yogic authenticity.

Niyama: Purifying Ourselves

There are five niyamas, or individual ethical observances. They are cleanliness (*sauca*), contentment (*santosa*), sustained practice (*tapas*), self-study (*svadhyaya*), and humble surrender to God (*Isvara pranidhana*). Sauca is related to the cleanliness achieved through asana practice. The cultivation of contentment (santosa) is to make the mind a fit instrument for meditation as contentment is the seed of the meditative state. Tapas is sustained practice, performed with passion, dedication, and devotion in order to gain physical prowess (*sakti*). Self-study, (svadhyaya) is the pursuit of skilful intelligence (*kushalata*). In action this is called *yukti,* which is the cleverness and clarity that are needed to follow the sadhana. Where self-study and self-knowledge are concerned, it is the petals of *pratyahara* (the inward investment of our energies) and *dharana* (concentration), which play the major role. Isvara pranidhana is *bhakti,* which means *total* surrender to God. Such surrender can only be the culmination of physical prowess and skilful intelligence. This is where the two petals of *dhyana* (meditation) and samadhi (blissful absorption) unite.

I should note here that *Isvara* is God in the universal, comprehensive sense, entirely cognate to the God of monotheistic religions. Isvara subsumes and includes all other concepts of divinity whatever their form or gender. It is just God, which is why I say that although Hindus have seemingly many gods, ultimately all combine in one monotheistic concept of the Supreme Being. Hindus are not idolaters, but people who worship the One in many forms, rather in the way that Christians might pray to a particular saint in relation to a specific problem.

It is a long journey from taking a bath to meeting God, so let us first look at how and why most of us remain stuck in the first two niyama.

Purity and Cleanliness

We can wash the skin of our bodies with a bath, but through asana practice we not only purify our blood and nourish cells. We are cleansing the inner body as we practice. By watching what we ingest into our bodies, we can keep our bodies cleaner. Geography has much to do with diet. Climate and other factors influence the diet people eat. But there are some basic guidelines that can help everyone. Do not eat if saliva does not spring from the mouth when food is brought before you. Secondly when the brain alone speculates about the choice of food, it means that the body does not need food. Even then, if you eat, it will be non-nourishing. It will be an abuse of food and will lead to overeating, which creates pollution in the body.

The subtle sheaths can also be cleansed. As we stop watching pornography and violence and stop having nightmares and become more self-aware, then the mind is cleansed, the lens of consciousness is cleaner, and this leads on axiomatically to the second niyama, which is contentment because contentment can only come from the ability to harmonize with our immediate environment.

Generally, what upsets us, what disturbs us, what makes us unhappy, is the everyday trivia like being growled at by the boss, having a row with one's spouse, failing an exam, or having a minor car accident. All these little things that happen in our immediate environment throw us off balance. A pure mind is a harmonious mind. Harmony exists both inwardly and outwardly. When consciousness, strength, and energy coordinate, then the little upsets of the day can be taken in our stride, dealt with for what they are—real but limited—and then put down. Contentment, which is an acceptance of one's mixed lot as a human being, returns. Resentment does not fester and poison even the satisfactory sections of our day.

If we have cleanliness and serenity inside, we can harmonize with the immediate environment. We're in balance and clean, so changes, disturbances, and events in our daily life do not throw us off balance. We can adapt to them. We're sensitive to them, we're flexible, we survive without trauma. You have a little accident with the car, but you realize it's no big deal, because you are flexible, you adapt.

This ability to harmonize with the immediate environment is a big payoff. From cleansing ourselves we have the contentment that comes from functioning in a smooth way with our environment and not being disturbed by its inevitable challenges and disturbances. That is the contentment of niyama and leads us on to being able to tackle the deeper levels of self-penetration and self-transformation. Because if we want to transform ourselves, we have to clean or purify, to have that serenity, flexibility, buoyancy within, and then we can go on to the transformations in the deeper levels of consciousness that are the yogic quest.

Most people practice yoga within the parameters of the first and second niyama, which are cleanliness and contentment. They get the immediate payoff of yoga practice (going to a class, doing a bit at home) from the fact that there is increasing health, which is cleanliness, and a deep health, an organic health, a mental clarity, well-being and repose, an ability to relax and rest, to nourish themselves from better breathing. So this brings an improvement in cleanliness, in deep health and concomitantly there is a greater contentment, integration with the environment, in our ability to handle its ups and downs. These are the two circles in which most people are living yoga. It is a quick and wonderful reward. Why then is it not enough just to stay with that since it is the definition of a good life decently and happily lived? Often if you don't carry on, if you settle for transient well-being, then new problems will arise. That is to say that when you are decently happy and clean and content then self-satisfaction will creep in. "I'm alright." This may lead to vanity and pride, a sort of smug superiority that is the dawning again of the intellectual defects that disfigure us. Or it may lead to lethargy and sluggishness, as we become complacent in our practice.

We are creatures that are designed for continual challenge. We must grow, or we begin to die. The status quo leads to stagnation and discontent. So just standing still isn't really an option. We have to move on. If not, disturbances will come. We've learned how to handle the disturbances of getting fired from our job, the outward ones, but when vanity and pride and smugness dawn, these disturbances, what I would call the diseases of the mind, take root within us. So nature offers us a new challenge. We're handling the day-to-day problems, but are we handling the inner disease of the growth of vanity, pride, and smugness in ourselves? This is a new challenge. We have to deal with it, but we won't if we get caught up in yoga for pleasure, the self-regarding yoga of saying, "I'm alright, aren't you in a mess." So the need to persevere derives from the fact that if we don't go further, new problems arise in which we become bogged down. That is why we are compelled to continue our practice.

The third, fourth, and fifth steps of niyama form a unit. The first is tapas, zealous, sustained practice that is at the heart of all yoga. I have repeatedly referred to tapas in earlier chapters as it is the thread that holds together the whole of yoga practice. It is literally heat, the heat that, in an alchemical sense, transforms. It is the practice that can never be abandoned, a continued application to human evolution.

Without the severe and penetrating insight of self-knowledge (svadhyaya), the fourth niyama, tapas would lead to power but neither penetration nor integration. It would merely generate energy but without direction. Tapas gives us the energy, svadhyaya the light of knowledge. Self-study is clearly intended to penetrate inward, and so the transforming fire of tapas enters progressively our different sheaths of being and illuminates us with self-knowledge. Self-knowledge may begin with recognizing the difficulty we have in controlling our desire for ice cream, but in deeper realms it concerns our duplicity, self-seeking, lust for power, desire for admiration, arrogance, and ultimately our wish to set ourselves up in the place of immortal God. Self-knowledge is not always comfortable. If we do not like what we find, we are, in all honesty, obliged to do something to alter it.

The fifth niyama is Isvara pranidhana, which means devotional surrender to God. This is the most theistic of all aspects of yoga. Isvara is Divinity in a general and nondenominational sense. What it definitely does not mean is using the ego to second-guess the will of God. It is, on the contrary, the surrender, through meditation (dhyana) and devotion (bhakti), of the ego itself. It is the absolute abandonment of the personal self. Therefore, personal ideas about what God may or may not want do not enter into the equation. It is offering oneself and all one's actions, however trivial, from cooking a meal to lighting a candle, to the Universal Divine. What the intentions of that Divinity may or may not be is not our business. All we have to do is revere the pristine, original, and eternal unity. God exists. It is this existence that illuminates our actions. That is surrender and devotion to the Supreme Being (Isvara pranidhana).

The niyama help us to establish a correct procedure and destroy the seeds of the afflictions (*dosabija*). Let us now look at the five niyama and integrate them more closely with the five sheaths of being and the rest of the eight petals of yoga. It is the practice of the yamas, niyamas, and six other petals of yoga that make possible the penetration from the skin to the soul.

Cleanliness as we have seen is more than having a bath. It is earned through the practice of asana that cleans both our inner and outer bodies. Cleanliness (sauca) is earned through the practice of asana and conquers the outer dominant inertia of the body and then infuses it with the vibrancy of *rajas*, providing a springboard to the higher qualities of life.

Contentment (santosa), in the yogic sense of lasting and stable harmony, is encountered through the practice of *pranayama*, which conquers in its turn the active (rajasic) nature of the mind and makes possible a practice that is both zealous and sustained. In santosa, the torso is a vessel that becomes filled with cosmic energy entering in the form of inhalation. Something, somewhere within us, makes room for cosmic energy, the bearer of cosmic intelligence, to take its place and install itself. This feels like something good or auspicious moving in. But in fact this is where evolution and involution marry. For the benevolence of contentment is equally the soul moving out from the center of being to occupy the torso. We are filling ourselves from outside, yes, but at this point, what is inside, being no longer blocked, moves out to fill us equally. This is the contentment of fullness, of the replete, but, at the out-breath, the soul expands to fill the space left by the breath and imbues us with a contentment that is not charged with *pranic* energy, but with soul's insight. Although the alternating state is dual, it quiets and nullifies the waves of the fluctuations of mind. In practical terms, it means that when something happens, I am not thrown off course, and when nothing happens, I do not lose my way.

The third niyama, tapas, sustained practice, corresponds to pratyahara, the hinge between the outer and inner aspects of yoga practice. It implies that cognitive awareness is bent inward with a view to self-knowledge (svadhyaya). It directs one toward the core of being and, like the blacksmith's bellows, it must always continue to heat the heart of the fire of practice, otherwise the alchemical transformation through extreme heat will never take place. The fire will burn merrily, but it will not turn lead into gold.

The fourth niyama, svadhyaya or self-knowledge, is difficult. We so much associate knowledge with the acquisition of learning (vidya). In reality, svadhyaya, whether through study or self-analysis, is the path of concentration (dharana), leading up a cruel and stony path to knowledge and to disrobing of the false or pretentious self with all its flaws and bogus virtues. Its reward is the path of wisdom, (*jnana marga*), which so denudes us of self-illusion that we are ready for the next great step.

This is surrender to God (Isvara pranidhana), often equated with bhakti, the yoga of supreme devotion and selflessness. Ego is on an elastic and will always pull you back. Only the practice of meditation will eventually erode the attraction between ego and self-identity.

Surrender to God is possible only for one who has, perhaps by circumstance or adversity or humiliation, discarded ego. For the surrender to be lasting, meditation in its highest sense must be accomplished. Surrender to God is not surrender to what you think God wants. It is not surrender to your conception of the will of God. It is not God giving you instructions. As long as ego persists, your interpretation of God's wishes will be fragmented by the distorting prism of ego. Only in an egoless state, that is the state of one who has attained the heights of seedless (*nirbija*) *samadhi*, will God's voice speak without an intervening screen of human frailty. And what will God tell you to do in this state of absolute freedom, of kaivalya? He will tell you to carry on in the world, but never to forget Him.

There is a story of a monk who strove for many years for emancipation. Despairing of ever reaching it, in spite of all his practices, he decided to climb the mountain next to his home, and there either to perish or to find illumination. He put his few goods in a backpack and set off up the mountain. Near the summit he met an old man coming down the mountain. Their eyes locked, and illumination took place. The monk's sack dropped to the ground. After moments of blissful silence, the monk looked at the old man and asked, "And now what shall I do?" Without words, the old man indicated the sack, signaled for him to shoulder it again and pointed back down the valley. The monk picked up his pack and went back down the valley. That was illumination on the mountain. What followed was kaivalya down in the valley.

I too live in the valley, in order to serve the needs of my students. I live in yogic practice (sadhana) in contact always with *asmita*, the subtle and individual "I" that is devoid of the growth of ego or pride. I am also a *hatha yogi*, which means I want my students to see the sun, to experience their own sun, their own soul. My students call me their guru. *Gu* means darkness and *ru* means light. My course as a sannyasin might have taken me into total reclusion, but I still feel it is my duty to serve, to be a guru in the sense of replacing the darkness with light. This is my dharma, my enduring duty. I have to be content with the divine restlessness that drives me on.

When I was young, I wanted to be an artist in my yoga practice. On first seeing the beautiful hands of Yehudi Menhuin, I thought, "I want artist's hands of such quality as that, rather than my coarse ones." I developed them to an incredible degree of sensitivity. But the motivation was not only yogic but also artistic. This impulse also fired my performances and my enjoyment of their reception. As a young, lost man, I was partly aspiring to artistry, partly to the yogic search for the soul. The one encouraged the other. Then pure yoga took me over, and artistry became secondary or incidental.

Life Is Learning

This whole book has been founded on a series of demarcations—the five sheaths, the five elements, their five subtle counterparts. It is a fruitful way to direct the quest toward the exploration of Nature and the discovery of the Soul. But in the back of our minds we should not forget that all sheaths and elements, all obvious demarcations, whether between gross or subtle bodies, do not arise at all. All are interwoven in consciousness. Hence the ultimate reach of yoga is the total transformation of citta (consciousness) that pervades our whole being with awareness and that knows no frontiers.

My hope is to have overcome the prejudice that Hatha Yoga is only physical and that it has nothing to do with the spiritual life. People have equated the practice of asana with physical practice. My life's work has been to show how, even from humble beginnings, this is a path that can lead the dedicated practitioner to the integration of body, mind, and soul.

What I have endeavored to say about asana is that the posture should be comfortable and steady. The steadiness comes only when the effort has ended. So you have to train the body in such a way that what seems complex becomes simple. In my asanas, I have no strain anywhere as my effort ceased long ago. Because my effort is at an end, I can offer my practice as an offering to the Lord God so that, in my practice, I join Him in the infinite.

We are wrong to think that we are all dull and inert. If your fire were extinguished, you would not be alive. Yogic fire (*yogagni*) exists in a latent or pristine state in everyone. It has consumed my life. But nothing is accomplished forever. If I let cool ashes cover my fire through carelessness, arrogance, or laxity of practice, the fire will lose its transforming heat. I have not retired and never shall. I will always keep the inner fire burning.

That is why practice (sadhana) cannot be stopped. Of course I age and regress at certain levels. But my body and mind are the servers and followers of the soul. The unity of these three gives me the right to call myself a yogi. But even though I am on a spiritual level, I will never say that practice is not required.

I am old, and death inevitably approaches. But both birth and death are beyond the will of a human being. They are not my domain. I do not think about it. Yoga has taught me to think of only working to live a useful life. The complexity of the life of the mind comes to an end at death, with all its sadness and happiness. If one is already free from that complexity, death comes naturally and smoothly. If you live holistically at every moment, as yoga teaches, even though the ego is annihilated, I will not say, "Die before you die." I would rather say, "Live before you die, so that death is also a lively celebration."

Hokkusei, the great Japanese artist, said when he was already in his seventies, that given another ten years, he would be a great artist. I salute his humility. Let me conclude by quoting the words of the Spanish artist Goya who, in the seventy-eighth year of his life, when he was already deaf and debilitated, said, *Aún aprendo*—"I am still learning." It is true for me too. I will never stop learning, and I have tried to share some of these lessons with you. I do pray that my ending will be your beginning. The great rewards and the countless blessings of a life spent following the Inward Journey await you.

Asanas for Emotional Stability

The following asanas will help you to develop emotional stability. When the given sequence is followed, they relax a person totally. The arrows show the right direction to extend and expand in the asana. For detailed step-by-step directions on how to perform each asana, please see my earlier book, *Light on Yoga*. I also recommend that you learn the practice under the guidance of an experienced and qualified teacher. It is important to do the practices correctly and precisely to receive the desired benefits and to avoid any harm.

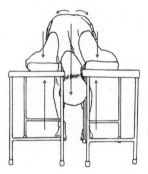

1. *Adho Mukha Svanasana*
(resting the head on support):
Stay for 2 to 3 minutes.

2. *Uttanasana* (resting the
head on the chair and head down
with the shoulders resting on two
high stools): Stay for 3 to 5 minutes.

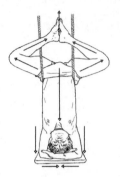

3. *Shirsasana* (using ropes):
Stay as long as you feel
comfortable.

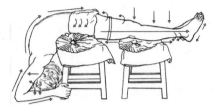

4. *Viparita Dandasana*
(on two stools):
Stay for 3 to 5 minutes.

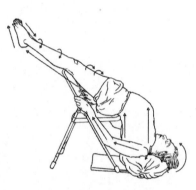

5. *Sarvangasana* (on a chair):
Stay for 5 to 10 minutes.

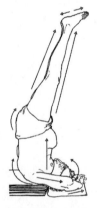

6. *Niralamba Sarvangasana*
(resting the shoulders on support):
Stay for 5 minutes.

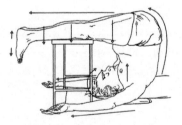

7. *Niralamba Halasana* (knees
or thighs resting on a stool):
Stay for 5 to 10 minutes.

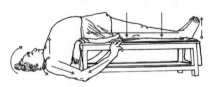

8. *Setubandha Sarvangasana*
(on a bench): Stay for 10 minutes.

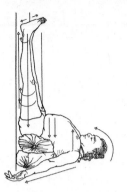

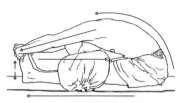

9. *Viparita Karani* in *Sarvangasana*
(here shown resting on two
bolsters): Stay for 5 minutes.

10. *Paschimottanasana* (head
resting on a bolster): Stay
for 3 to 5 minutes.

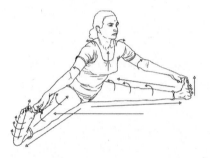

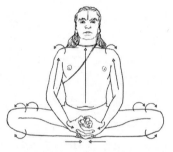

11. *Upavista Konasana*: (If one cannot hold the toes, one can sit straight
with palms on the floor behind
the buttocks.) Stay for 2 minutes.

12. *Baddhakonasana*: (Roll a
blanket and place underneath
the knees for comfort.) Stay
for 3 to 5 minutes.

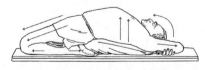

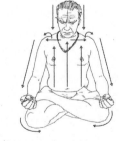

13. *Supta Virasana* (on a bolster):
Stay as long as you can lie
with ease.

14. *Viloma Pranayama* (with interrupted exhalation either in sitting
or lying position): If done in sitting
position, stay for 5 to 8 minutes.

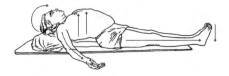

15. *Shavasana* with chest elevated: (Some bolsters or a heavy weight to be kept on the thighs for a quick relaxation of the body and a wrapped cloth around the eyes for the relaxation of the brain. The weight on the thighs opens the lungs.) This can be done at any time, even after meals, according to one's available time.

Please note:

While doing *Sarvangasana* on the chair (5), if you feel pressure on the temples, you can instead do *Niralamba Sarvangasana* (6). *Sarvangasana* on the chair can be tried after doing *Niralamba Sarvangasana* first in the beginning.

Niralamba Sarvangasana (6), *Setubandha Sarvangasana* on a bench (8), and *Viparita Karani* in *Sarvangasana* (9) are very good for those suffering from migraine.

- Asanas 1 to 3 completed in sequence of asanas calms the mind and cools the brain.
- Asanas 4 to 10 balance the intelligence of the head (intellectual center) and the intelligence of the heart (emotional center).
- Asanas 11 and 12 stimulate the brain for positive thinking.
- Asana 13 brings quietness in the body.
- Asana 14 allows you to experience inner silence.
- If you do not have enough time, skip asana 14 and go to 15. If time allows, do for 5 to 10 minutes.

Index

Boldface page references indicate photographs.

A

Abhinivesa. *See* Fear of Death or
    Clinging to Life
Abhyasa (practice), 93–94, 99–100,
    102–3, 112
Action
    complementary, 43
    direct, 137
    intelligence and, 28
    precision in, 42
    silence and, 31–32
    teaching and, 221
    types of, 247
Adam and Eve, 170–71
Addictions, 96, 143, 169
Adho Mukha Svanasana (resting head
    on support), 267, **267**
Afflictions (klesa)
    Attachment, 195–96, 199–200
    Aversion, 195–97
    concept of, 190–91
    Fear of Death or Clinging to Life,
        197–99, 256–57
    Ignorance, 191–93, 199
    interference of, 151
    Inward Journey and, 199–200
    mastering, 256–57
    Pride, 194–95
Aggression, 41–42
Ahamkara (I-shape), 111–13, 117–22,
    124
Ahamkara (small self), 111, 117–22,
    215
Ahimsa (nonviolence), 251–52
AIDS epidemic, 116
Aims of Life (Purusartha), 237–41
Aloneness, 184
Analysis (vitarka), 39, 154
Anandamaya kosa. *See* Divine body;
    Sheaths of being
Anger, 88–90, 135
Annamaya kosa. *See* Physical body;
    Sheaths of being
Antahkarana (conscience), 101,
    178–80, 250

Antara kumbhaka (retention of breath
    after inhalation), 72, 75, 77, 93,
    184–85
Aparigrahah (non-covetousness or
    modesty of life), 254
Architecture, 203
Ardha chandrasana (half-moon asana
    pose), 141
Arrogance, 194–96
Artha (self-reliance of earning own
    living), 237–39
Art (kala), 204
Asanas. *See* Postures of yoga
Ascension, final, 201–7
Ashrama (Stages of Life), xiii, 241–46
Asmita (I-am-ness), 120, 122, 188–90
Asmita (pride), 87–88, 194–95
Asteya (non-stealing), 253–54
Atma. *See* Soul
Attachment (raga), 195–96, 199–200
Aum Namo Narayanaya ("seed
    prayer"), 252
Aurobindo, 170
Aversion (dvesa), 195–97
Avidya (Ignorance), 121–22, 191–93, 199
Awareness (prajna), 171
    balance of, 42
    consciousness and, 145
    cosmic, 149
    intellectual body and, 155, 162–65
    meditation and, 15
    mind and, 155
    physical body and, 28–33

B

Baddhakonasana pose, 269, **269**
Bahya kumbhaka (retention of breath
    after exhalation), 72, 76, 93,
    184–85
Balance
    of awareness, 42
    of elements, 206
    life and, 44
    physical body and, 25, 42–47
    of sheaths of being, 4–6, 103

Behavioral patterns, altering embedded, 131–38, 141–42
Bhakti (devotion), 212
Bhogakala (art of appeasing the pleasure of body and mind), 204
Bhoga yoga (proficient complacency), 58
Bhumis (Five Qualities of Mind), 165–66
Black holes, 213–14
Bliss. *See* Divine body
Bondage, 93
Brahmacarya (continence or celibacy), 254–55
Brahmacaryasrama (first stage of life), 241–42
Brahman (God), 8, 59, 65–66, 205, 249–50, 263–64
Breathing technique (pranayama)
    calming emotions and, 96–97
    concentration and, 72, 183–84
    consciousness and, 93
    contentment and, 262
    exhalation, 72, 75–76, 97–98, 184–85
    fear and, liberating, 104
    Fear of Death and, 104–5
    fire element and, 71
    inhalation, 72, 74–75
    introversion and, 73
    lung capacity and, 69–70
    meditation and, 183–84
    mind and, 75–77
    parts of yogic, 72
    in petals of yoga, 10, 12
    physical movements of, 74–76
    retention of breath after exhalation, 72, 76, 93, 184–85
    retention of breath after inhalation, 72, 75, 77, 93, 184–85
    water element and, 71
Bridge pose (Setu Bandha Sarvangasana), 81

C

Celibacy (brahmacarya), 254–55
Cellular level of memory, 144–45
Challenges of life, xiii–xiv, 260–61
Change, process of, 160–61

Chidra citta (imperfect consciousness), 221
Chi (life energy), 65
Citta. *See* Consciousness
Clarity. *See* Mental body
Cleanliness (sauca), 257–65
Cleverness, 230–31, 258
Clinging to Life. *See* Fear of Death or Clinging to Life
Cognition, 126–27, 152
Communication, 83, 120
Compassion, 19, 52, 95–96
Conation, 127
Concentration (dharana)
    breathing technique and, 72, 183–84
    intellectual body and, 180–82
    intelligence and, 176
    in petals of yoga, 10, 13–14
    steadiness of mind and, 98
    wisdom and, 103
Conscience (antahkarana), 101, 178–80, 250
Consciousness (citta)
    awareness and, 145
    breathing technique and, 93
    cosmic intelligence and, 208
    disease and, 24
    energy body and, 68, 76–77, 102
    Five Modifications of, 153–54
    fluctuations in, 131–32, 147
    forms of, 153–54
    functions of, 152
    Healthy and Healing Qualities of, 94–99, 153–54
    imperfect, 221
    inner workings of, 110–13
    intellectual body and, 151–52
    intelligence and, 68, 145
    mental body and, 110–13, 124
    microcosmic level of, 198
    mind and, 198
    parts of, 111
    transformations of, 220
    true ethics and, 250
    universal, 169
    vital energy and, 102
    yoga and, 109, 111, 220
Contemplation, 98

Contentment (santosa), 257, 259, 262
Continence (brahmacarya), 254–55
Corpse pose (Savasana), 159, 232–37
Correct knowledge (pramana), 153, 161
Cosmic awareness, 149
Cosmic Divine, 97
Cosmic game (lila), 206
Cosmic intelligence (mahat), 68, 149,
    172–73, 207–8, 213
Cosmic Soul, 201
Courage (virya), 94
Creative potential, xxi

D

Darsan (philosophy), 110–12, 125
Darwin, Charles, 208
DaVinci, Leonardo, 41
Death. *See* Fear of Death or Clinging
    to Life
Deduction, 161
Density, 45
Detachment (vairagya), 93–94, 99,
    244–45
Determination (drdhata), 94
Devotion (bhakti), 212
Dharana. *See* Concentration
Dharma (spiritual values), 192–93, 237,
    240–41
Dharmendriya (organ of virtue), 101
Dhyana. *See* Meditation
Dilemmas, 53–54
Discernment, 113, 123–31
Discretion (vivecana), 93
Discrimination (viveka), 93, 155, 162,
    230
Disease, 23–24, 52, 115–16
Divine body (anandamaya kosa). *See
    also* Sheaths of being
  Afflictions and
    Attachment, 195–96, 199–200
    Aversion, 195–97
    concept of, 190–91
    Fear of Death or Clinging to Life,
      197–99, 256–57
    Ignorance, 191–93, 199
    interference of, 151
    Inward Journey and, 199–200
    Pride, 194–95

Ascension and, final, 201–7
balancing, with other kosas, 4–6
concept of, 187–90
coordination of, with other kosas,
    27–28, 103
evolution of Nature and, 207–10
"I" concept and, 187–90
meditation and, 200–201
physical body and, 205
union and, 214–25
yoga as involution and, 211–14
Divine Will, 201
Drdhata (determination), 94
Duality, 16, 44–45, 207
Dvesa (aversion), 195–97
Dynamic extension, 33–38
Dynamism (rajas), 45, 207

E

Ears, 73
Earth, 6–9, 205
Echo exhalation, 97
Ego, 36, 87, 91, 120–21, 136, 180, 185,
    198
Elements, 71, 206
Emotional Disturbances
  anger, 88–90
  greed, 91–93
  hatred, 90–91
  lust, 85–87
  managing, 81–82
  obsession, 87–88
  overview, 82–85
  pride, 87–88
Emotional stability, asanas for, 267–70,
    267–70
Emotions, 85, 96–97. *See also*
    Emotional Disturbances
Endurance, 48
Energy body (pranamaya kosa). *See also*
    Breathing technique; Sheaths
    of being
  balancing, with other kosas, 4–6
  breath and, 69–77
  concept of, 65–68
  consciousness and, 68, 76–77, 102
  coordination of, with other kosas,
    27–28, 103

Energy body *(cont.)*
  cosmic intelligence and, 208, 213
  Emotional Disturbances and
    anger, 88–90
    greed, 91–93
    hatred, 90–91
    lust, 85–87
    managing, 81–82
    obsession, 87–88
    overview, 82–85
    pride, 87–88
  enjoyment and, 93–94
  Healthy and Healing Qualities of
    Consciousness and, 94–99
  humility and, 73
  intelligence and, 68
  Inward Journey and, 67–68
  mind and, 75–77
  paradox of, 213–14
  Patanjali and, 67
  physical body and, 68
  physical movements of, 74–76
  sensory control and withdrawal and,
    99–105
  stress and, 77–82
Enjoyment, 93–94
Erasmus, 192
Erroneous knowledge, 159–60
Ethics
  vs. morals, 248
  personal, 246–50
  true, 10, 176, 247, 250–57
  universal, 246–50
Evolution of Nature, 207–10
Exhalation (recaka), 72, 75–76, 97–98,
  184–85
Extroversion, 73
Eyes, 38–39, 73, 205

F

Faith (sraddha), 94
Fantasy (vikalpa), 153, 156–57, 201
Fear of Death or Clinging to Life
  (abhinivesa)
  as Affliction, 197–200, 256–57
  breathing technique and, 104–5
  I-consciousness and, 121–22
Feeling, 85

Final Ascension, 201–7
Final integration. *See* Union
Fire element, 71
Freedom (moksa)
  achieving, 170
  to adolescent, 243–44
  Aims of Life and, 237–41
  to children, 243–44
  cleanliness and, 258–65
  dynamic extension and, 36
  economic, 227
  eternal, 224–25, 228
  ethics and
    personal, 246–50
    true, 247, 250–57
    universal, 246–50
  Inward Journey and, xxii, 11
  learning and, 265–66
  living in, 237–41
  memory and, 138–46
  pain and, 48
  political, 227
  power and, 173, 230–31
  self-purification and, 257–58
  space and, 202–5
  spiritual, 227
  Stages of Life and, 241–46
  union and, 228–30
Free Will, 168–69

G

Gandhi, Mahatma, xxi, 16, 157, 170
Gandhiji, 96, 251–52
Gaudi, 203–4
God (Brahman), 8, 59, 65–66, 205,
  249–50, 263–64
Goya, 266
Gratitude, 195–96
Greed, 91–93
Grhasthsrama (second stage of life),
  242–44
Gunas, 44–47, 207

H

Habits, giving up bad (samskara),
  131–38, 141–42
Halasana (plough pose), 81

Half-moon asana pose (ardha
chandrasana), 141
Hanuman asana pose, 50
Happiness, 52, 93–94, 95
Harmony, 42–47, 63, 259. *See also*
Balance
Hatha Yoga, 151
Hatha Yoga Pradipika, 76–77
Hatred, 90–91
Hawking, Stephen, 213
Health, 23–28, 171
Healthy and Healing Qualities of
Consciousness (citta vrittis),
94–99, 153–54
High intelligence, 177
Hokkusei, 266
Holy Grail, 3
Horizontal dynamic extension, 35–36
Hubris, 87–88, 194–96
Human being as continuum, 6
Humility, 73

I

I-am-ness (asmita), 120, 122, 188–90.
See also Pride
I-awareness, 121–22
"I" concept, 187–90
I-consciousness, 120–22, 158
Ignorance (avidya), 121–22, 191–93, 199
Illness, 23–24, 52, 115–16
Imagination (vikalpa), 153, 156–57, 201
Impurities, 25, 97, 174–78
Individuality, 76
Individual soul (jivatman), 148, 178,
185, 200
Inertia (tamas), 45, 183, 207
Infinite, 44–45, 202, 204
Inhalation (puraka), 72, 74–75
Innovation, 123
In Praise of Folly (Erasmus), 192
Insight, 162–65
Instinct, 163
Integration, xiv, 224–25. *See also* Union
Integrity, 86
Intellectual body (vijnanamaya kosa).
See also Sheaths of being
awareness and, 155, 162–65
balancing, with other kosas, 4–6

bhumis and, 165–66
concentration and, 180–82
concept of, 147–49
conscience and, 178–80
consciousness and, 151–52
coordination of, with other kosas,
27–28, 103
insight and, 162–65
intelligence and
culture of, 166–71
examining, 149–51
impurities of, 174–78
lens analogy and, 151–52
intuition and, 162–65
meditation and, 182–86
mental body and, 108, 147
mind and, 152–61
physical body and, 39
physical prowess and, 171–73
power and, 171–73
proof and, 161–62
Intellectual skills (yukti), 212
Intelligence. *See also* Wisdom
achievements of, 175–76
action and, 28
awakening, 128
characteristics of, 123–24
cognition and, 126
concentration and, 176
conscience and, 178–80
consciousness and, 68, 145
cosmic, 68, 149, 172–73, 207–8,
213
culture of, 166–71
discernment and, 113, 123–31
discrimination and, 155
energy body and, 68
examining, 149–51
high, 177
impurities of, 148, 174–78
intellectual body and
culture of, 166–71
examining, 149–51
impurities of, 174–78
lens analogy and, 151–52
knowledge of body and, 49
lens analogy and, 151–52
memory and, 143–44, 177
mental body and, 123–31

Intelligence (cont.)
  mind and, 155–56
  mirror of, 125
  physical body and, 28–29
  postures of yoga and, 162
  skillful, 257
  universal, 68
  will and, 126–27
  wisdom and, 164–65
Introspection, 73
Introversion, 73
Intuition, 162–65
Invention, 123
Involution, 102, 211–14
Inward Journey. See also Yoga
  Afflictions and, 199–200
  concept of, 173
  embarking on, ix, xiv
  energy body and, 67–68
  freedom and, xxii, 11
  learning and, 266
  Nature and
    elements of, 6–9
    living with, 18–19
    Universal Soul and, 9–10
  nature of, 18–19
  personal experience of, ix-xii, xvi-xx
  petals of yoga
    breathing technique, 10, 12
    concentration, 10, 13–14
    meditation, 10, 13–16
    postures, 10–12
    self-purification, 10–11
    sensory control and withdrawal,
      10, 12–13
    sheaths of being and, 10
    union, 10, 13, 17–18
    universal moral commandments, 10
  role models for, ix
  self-knowledge and, xxi-xxii, 3
  sheaths of being and, 4–6
I-shape (ahamkara), 111–13, 117–22, 124
Isvara pranidhana, 258, 261, 263

J

Jesus, 170
Jivatman (individual soul), 148, 178,
  185, 200

Jnana. See Intellectual body; Wisdom
Joy, 52, 93–94, 95

K

Kaivalya (eternal freedom), 224–25,
  228
Kaivalya Pada (the Freedom Chapter),
  227–28
Kala (art), 204
Kama (pleasures of love and human
  enjoyment), 237
Karma, 136–37, 209, 221
Karuna (cultivation of passion), 95
Ki (life energy), 65
Klesa. See Afflictions
Knowledge, 153, 159–60, 161–62. See
  also Self-knowledge
Kosas. See Sheaths of being
Kundalini energy, 89–90, 222–23
Kushalata (skillful intelligence), 257

L

Lao Tzu, 117
Learning, 59, 265–66
Life
  Aims of, 237–41
  balance and, 44
  challenges of, xiii-xiv, 260–61
  dilemmas in, 53–54
  energy, 65
  learning and, 265–66
  Soul and, 137–38
  Stages of, xiii, 241–46
  stress in, 78, 80
  wholeness in, xiv, 194
  yoga and, xvi, xx-xxii, 22
Light, quality of (sattva), 45, 207
Lightness and physical body, 40–42, 49
Light on the Yoga Sutras of Patanjali
  (Iyengar), xi
Lila (cosmic game), 206
Loneliness, 184
Love
  divine, 85–86
  physical body and, 59
  sensual desire and, 86–87
  sexual, 254–55

Luminosity (sattva), 45, 207
Lung capacity, 69–70. *See also*
    Breathing technique
Lust, 85–87

M

Maharishi, Ramana, 70
Mahat (cosmic intelligence), 68, 149,
    172–73, 207–8, 213
Maitri (cultivation of friendliness), 94–95
Manolaya, 218
Manomaya kosa. *See* Mental body;
    Sheaths of being
Mass (tamas), 45, 183, 207
Meditation (dhyana)
    awareness and, 15
    breathing technique and, 183–84
    divine body and, 200–201
    intellectual body and, 182–86
    in petals of yoga, 10, 13–16
    in stress management, 80–81
    wisdom and, 15
    yoga and, 80–81, 94, 184
Memory (smrti)
    of body, 144
    cellular level of, 144–45
    cleansing, 156
    ego and, 120
    freedom and, 138–46
    imprints of, 145
    intelligence and, 143–44, 177
    liberation vs. bondage, 138–46, 154
    mental body and, 138–46
    mind and, 114, 144
    past and, 43–44
    perception and, 145–46
    physical body and, 57
    postures of yoga and, 57
    purifying, 156
Mental body (manomaya kosa). *See*
    also Sheaths of being
    balancing, with other kosas, 4–6
    concept of, 107–10
    consciousness and, 110–13, 124
    coordination of, with other kosas,
        27–28, 103
    habits and, giving up bad, 131–38,
        141–42

intellectual body and, 108, 147
intelligence and, 123–31
I-shape and, 117–22
memory and, 138–46
mind and, 113–17
Menuhin, Yehudi, 87–88, 264
Michelangelo, 180
Military training, 100
Mind. *See also* Mental body
    awareness and, 155
    breathing technique and, 75–77
    as computer, human, 113–17
    consciousness and, 198
    energy body and, 75–77
    Five Qualities of, 165–66
    fluctuating, 153–54
    innovation vs. invention and, 123
    intellectual body and, 152–61
    intelligence and, 155–56
    memory and, 114, 144
    mental body and, 113–17
    nature of, 152–53
    penetration of, 45–46
    states of inner, 220
    survival tool of, 114–15
    transforming, 152–61
    workings of, 128–30
    yoga and, 109
Mind-body connection, xv
Misconception (viparyaya), 153,
    164
Modesty of life (aparigrahah), 254
Moksa. *See* Freedom
Morals and morality, 248, 250, 252
Mother Teresa of Calcutta, 96
Motion, 152
Mountain pose (tadasana), 7, 108
Movement of skin, 33–36
Mudita (cultivation of joy), 95

N

Nature (Prakrti)
    elements of, 6–9
    evolution of, 207–10
    as initiating power, 62
    living with, 18–19
    physical body and, 22–23
    scientist and, 19

Nature *(cont.)*
  Soul and, 9–10, 170
  Universal Soul and, 9–10
  vacuum and, 204
  will and, 62
  yoga and, 207–9
  yogi and, 19
Newton, Isaac, 208
Nidra (sleep), 98–99, 153–54,
    157–59
Niralamba Halasana (knees or thighs
    resting on stool), 268, **268**
Niralamba Sarvangasana (shoulders
    resting on support), 268, **268**
Niyama (self-purification), 10–11, 140,
    176, 257–58, 261
Non-covetousness (aparigrahah), 254
Non-physical reality, 8
Non-stealing (asteya), 253–54
Nonviolence (ahimsa), 251–52

O

Obsession, 87–88
Oneness, xiv, 201. *See also* Union
Organ of virtue (dharmendriya), 101
Overstretching, 34
Ownership, 195–96

P

Pain
  freedom and, 48
  physical body and, 47–54
  pleasure and, 137
  right, 50–51
  wrong, 50–51
Paschimottanasana (head resting on
    bolster), 269, **269**
Passion, 85
Past, 43–44, 57
Patanjali, x–xi, 7, 27, 67, 94, 98, 101–2,
    108–9, 128, 150, 153, 156, 175,
    219–20, 227–28, 230, 238,
    249–50
Pavlov, Ivan, 138
Perception, 137, 145–46, 161
Perfection, 54–61, 236
Personal ethics, 246–50
Petals of yoga. *See* Yoga

Philosophy (darsan), 110–12, 125
Physical body (annamaya kosa). *See
    also* Postures of yoga; Sheaths
    of being
  aggression and, 41–42
  awareness and, 28–33
  balance and, 25, 42–47
  balancing, with other kosas, 4–6
  concept of, 21–23
  coordination of, with other kosas,
      27–28, 30, 103
  disease and, 23
  divine body and, 205
  dynamic extension and, 33–38
  earth and, 205
  endurance and, 48
  energy body and, 68
  exertion of, 45–46
  guana and, 44–47
  health and, 23–28
  intellectual body and, 39
  intelligence and, 28–29
  lightness of, 40–42, 49
  love and, 59
  memory and, 57
  movement of skin and, 33–36
  Nature and, 22–23
  pain and, 47–54
  Patanjali's definition of, 27
  penetration of mind and, 45–46
  Perfection and, 54–61
  postures of yoga and, 61–64
  relaxation and, 36–40
  rigid, 41–42
  soft, 41
  soul and, 22–23
  stretching and, 33–38
  value of, 24
  yoga and, 22, 30
Physical prowess (sakti), 171–73, 212,
    257
Pleasure, 137, 175
Plough pose (halasana), 81
Poses or positions of yoga. *See* Postures
    of yoga
Positive emotions, 96
Postures of yoga
  bridge pose, 81
  corpse pose, 159, 232–37

for emotional stability, 267–70,
   267–70
half-moon asana pose, 141
hanuman asana pose, 50
intelligence and, 162
memory and, 57
mountain pose, 7, 108
personal experience with, xvi-xx
in petals of yoga, 10–12
physical body and, 61–64
plough pose, 81
practicing, 10–12, 55–56
purpose of, xvi
standing still and straight pose, 108
transformation of, in public eye, xiii
triangle pose, 61–62, 223
Power
  of awareness, 171
  ego and, 87
  freedom and, 173, 230–31
  of healthy body, 171
  intellectual body and, 171–73
  Nature as initiating, 62
  of pranic energy, 171
  siddhis and, 230
  of soul, 171
  types of, 171
  virtuous, 63
  wisdom and, 171–73
Practice (abhyasa), 93–94, 99–100,
  102–3, 112
Prajna. *See* Awareness
Prakrti. *See* Nature
Pramana (correct knowledge), 153
Pranamaya kosa. *See* Energy body;
  Sheaths of being
Prana sakti (power of pranic energy),
  171
Prana (vital energy), 102. *See also*
  Energy body
Pranayama. *See* Breathing technique
Pratyahara (sensory control and
  withdrawal)
  calming Emotional Disturbances and,
    99–105
  energy body and, 99–105
  in petals of yoga, 10, 12–13
Prerana, 169
Present (time), 44

Pride (asmita), 87–88, 194–95. *See also*
  I-am-ness
Proof, 161–62
Puraka (inhalation), 72, 74–75
Purity, 25–26, 258–65
Purusartha (Aims of Life), 237–41
Purusa (Self), 44, 62, 72, 170

R

Raga (attachment), 195–96, 199–200
Rage, 88–90, 135
Rajasic sleep, 158–59
Rajas (vibrancy or dynamism), 45, 207
Ramakrishna, 86, 218–19
Ramanujacharya, 252
Ramon, Ilan, 16
Reality
  of earth and sky, 6
  non-physical, 8
  Universal, 8–9
Reasoning (vicara), 93
Rebellion, 243–44
Recaka (exhalation), 72, 75–76, 97–98,
  184–85
Reflection, inner, 31
Relaxation, 36–40, 232–33
Repetition, 93
Retention of breath after exhalation
  (bahya kumbhaka), 72, 76, 93,
  184–85
Retention of breath after inhalation
  (antara kumbhaka), 72, 75, 77,
  93, 184–85
Revelation, 142
Rigidity, 25, 41–42
Rig Veda, 8–9
Rumination, 142

S

Sabija samadhi, 218
Sadhana, ix, 167–68
Sakti (physical prowess), 171–73, 212,
  257
Samadhi. *See* Union
Samasthiti (standing still and straight
  pose), 108
Samskara (giving up bad habits),
  131–38, 141–42

Sannyasin (fourth and final stage of
    life), xiii, 245–46
Santosa (contentment), 257, 259, 262
Sarira sakti (power of a healthy body), 171
Sarvangasana (on chair), 268, **268**
Sastra (science), 78, 204, 208
Sattva (luminosity or quality of light),
    45, 207
Sattva-suddhi, 128
Sattvic sleep, 158
Sauca (cleanliness), 257–65
Savasana (corpse pose), 159, 232–37
Science of religion, 237
Science (sastra), 78, 204, 208
Seer, xv, 137–38
self, small (ahamkara), 111, 117–22, 215
Self-awareness, 31
Self-consciousness, 31
Self-control, 81–82
Self-knowledge (svadhyaya), xxi-xxii, 3,
    102–3, 169, 175–76, 178
Self-purging, 59–60
Self-purification (niyama), 10–11, 140,
    176, 257–58, 261
Self (Purusa), 44, 62, 72, 170
Self-realization, ix, 251
Self-reliance of earning own living
    (artha), 237-39
Self-study (svadhyaya), 9, 94, 257–58,
    263
Sensitivity, 25–26, 33
Sensory control and withdrawal
    (pratyahara)
  calming Emotional Disturbances and,
      99–105
  energy body and, 99–105
  in petals of yoga, 10, 12–13
Sensual desire, 86–87
Setubandha Sarvangasana (bridge pose),
    81
Setubandha Sarvangasana (on bench),
    268, **268**
Sexuality, 87
Shakespeare, William, 87
Shavasana, 270, **270**
Sheaths of being (kosas). *See also*
    specific types
  balancing, 4–6, 103
  cleanliness and, 259

demarcation of different, 5
divine (anandamaya kosa), 4–6, 62,
    187, 205
energy (pranamaya kosa), 4–6, 64,
    68, 82, 103
integration of, final, xiv, 224–25
intelligence or wisdom (vijnanmaya
    kosa), 4–6, 39, 108, 147
Inward Journey and, 4–6
mental (manomaya kosa), 4–6, 103,
    108
petals of yoga and, 10
physical (annamaya kosa), 4–6,
    27–28, 30, 68, 103, 205
Shirsasana (using ropes), 268, **268**
Siddhis, 230
Silence, 31–32
Sistine Chapel, 180
Skin, sensitivity and movement of,
    33–36
Sky, 6–9
Sleep (nidra), 98–99, 153–54, 157–59
Smrti. *See* Memory
Socrates, xxi, 169
Soft emotions, 96
Soul (atma)
  conscience and, 179
  Cosmic, 201
  individual, 148, 178, 185, 200
  life and, 137–38
  Nature and, 9–10, 170
  physical body and, 22–23
  power of, 171
  as "third eye," 39
  Universal, 9–10
Space, 202–5
Spiritual realization, 3
Spiritual values (dharma), 192–93, 237,
    240–41
Sports, Western, 26–27
Sraddha (faith), 94
Stability. *See* Physical body
Stages of Life (Ashrama), xiii, 241–46
Standing still and straight pose
    (samasthiti), 108
Stevenson, George, 82–83
Stress
  energy body and, 77–82
  in life, 78, 80

meditation in managing, 80–81
yoga in managing, 79–80
Stretching, 33–38
Suffering, 52
Superiority, avoiding, 58
Supta Virasana (on bolster), 269, **269**
Surrender to God, 263–64
Survival, 114–15
Sustained practice (tapas), 94, 102–3,
    212, 257–58, 263
Suzuki, D.T., 247
Svadhyaya (self-study and self-
    knowledge), xxi-xxii, 3, 9, 94,
    102–3, 169, 175–76, 178, 212,
    257–58, 263
Svatmarama, 76
Synthesis (vicara), 39

T

Tadasana (mountain pose), 7, 108
Tamas (mass or inertia), 45, 183, 207
Tapas (sustained practice), 94, 102–3,
    212, 257–58, 263
Tasmasic sleep, 154, 158
Technology, 78
Temptation, 101–2
Testimony, 161
Throat, 38, 74
Time, 43–44, 57, 142, 232–37
Total abosorption. *See* Union
Toxins, 25
Triangle pose (Trikonasana), 61–62, 223
Truth, 19, 252–53, 257

U

Understretching, 34
Union (samadhi)
    concept of, 214–16
    divine body and, 214–25
    experience of, 186
    final integration of, xiv, 224–25
    freedom and, 228–30
    kaivalya and, 224–25
    kundalini energy and, 222–23
    manolaya and, 218
    in petals of yoga, 10, 13, 17–18
    physical basis of, 219–20

problems of, 217–18
Ramakrishna and, 86
reaching, 201
sabija samadhi and, 218
seeking, 223–24
self and, 215
sleep and, 158
state of, 215–17
Universal consciousness, 169
Universal ethics, 246–50
Universal intelligence, 68
Universal moral commandments
    (yama), 10, 176, 247, 250–57
Universal Reality, 8–9
Universal Soul, 9–10
Upavista Konasana, 269, **269**
Upeksa (cultivation of indifference), 95
Uttanasana (resting head on chair), 267,
    267

V

Vairagya (detachment), 93–94, 99,
    244–45
Vanaprasthasrama (third stage of life),
    244–45
Vertical ascending, 44
Vertical descending, 44
Vertical dynamic extension, 35–36
Vibrancy (rajas), 45, 207
Vibration, 205
Vicara (reasoning), 93
Vicara (synthesis), 39
Vijnanamaya kosa. *See* Intelligent body;
    Sheaths of being
Vikalpa (imagination or fantasy), 153,
    156–57, 201
Viloma Pranayama, 269, **269**
Viparita Dandasana (on two stools),
    268, **268**
Viparita Karani pose, 269, **269**
Viparyaya (wrong knowledge or
    misconception), 153, 164
Virtue, 86, 96, 101
Virya (courage), 94
Vishnu, 252
Vital energy, 102. *See also* Energy body
Vitarka (analysis), 39, 154
Vitruvius Man, 41

Vivecana (discretion), 93
Viveka (discrimination), 93, 155, 162, 230
Volition, 127, 152. *See also* Will

W

Waste of resources, 91
Water element, 71
Waves, 45, 131–32, 205
Western sports, 26–27
Wholeness in life, xiv, 194
Will (human), 14, 29, 56, 62, 126–27, 169
Willpower, 56
Wisdom (jnana). *See also* Intellectual body; Intelligence
  concentration and, 103
  intelligence and, 164–65
  meditation and, 15
  power and, 171–73
  yoga and, 203
Wrong knowledge (viparyaya), 153, 164

Y

Yama (universal moral commandments or true ethics), 10, 176, 247, 250–57
Yoga. *See also* Inward Journey; Poses of yoga
  art and science of, ix, 167–68
  benefits of, xxi
  bhoga, 58
  challenge of, 50
  consciousness and, 109, 111, 220
  creative potential and, xxi
  vs. Darwin, 208
  demands of, 21–22
  divine, 61–64
  eyes and, 38–39
  of final integration (samyama yoga), 10, 13, 17–18
  goal of, 11, 133–34
  gunas and, 46–47
  intensity of, 60–61
  as involution, 211–14

joy of, 26, 93–94
knowledge of, 94
life and, xvi, xx–xxii, 22
meditation and, 80–81, 94, 184
mind and, 109
mind-body connection and, xv
Nature and, 207–9
Newton and, 208
"Olympics," 27
perfection and, 236
perspective of, xv–xvi
petals of
  breathing technique, 10, 12
  concentration, 10, 13–14
  meditation, 10, 13–16
  posture, 10–12
  self-purification, 10–11
  sensory control and withdrawal, 10, 12–13
  sheaths of being and, 10
  union, 10, 13, 17–18
  universal moral commandments, 10
philosophy of, 110–12
physical body and, 22, 30
sadhana, 167–68
in stress management, 79–80
techniques of, 103–4
throat and, 38
transformation of, in public eye, xiii
as universal path, xiv–xv
value of, x
vs. Western sports, 26–27
wholeness in life and, xiv
will and, 169
wisdom of, 203
Yogagni (yogic fire), 265–66
Yogakala (art of auspicious performance to please spiritual heart of soul), 204
Yogasana. *See* Postures of yoga
Yoga Sutras (Patanjali), 7, 27, 108
Yogic fire (yogagni), 265–66
Yogic journey. *See* Inward Journey; Yoga
Yukti (intellectual skills), 212